AF175291

Marianne E. Meyer
Survival Aid for All Viral Infections
Guide for Perfect Immune Protection
Scalar Wave Analysis – Breakthrough in Medical Diagnostics

Produce and publishing
BoD - Books on Demand, Norderstedt
ISBN 978-3-756-212125

The information introduced in this book was carefully researched and imparted in all conscience. However, the author and publisher don't take any liability for damages of any nature emerging directly or indirectly from the use or application of this book's data. The data of this work is for interested parties and education.

Some other books by M. E. Meyer:

Spirulina – Survival Food for a New Era
How Water Connects our Worlds
Cranberry Power Fruit
Family Code
Beyond Death
Migrant Birds on Wheels

Cover design,
typesetting & layout: M. Meyer

Photo credit:
Thank you for providing the following pictorial material: M. Meyer, p. 8, 22, 28, 35, 42, 51,55, 62,63, M. Hagenaar, p. 11, 105, 108, Pflanzmich p. 39, S. de Jesus p. 58, J. Janzen p.77, R. Taylor p. 105
Cover: R. Taylor, M. Meyer

Marianne E. Meyer

Survival Aid for All Viral Infections

Guide for Perfect Immune Protection

Scalar Wave Analysis – Breakthrough in Medical Diagnostics

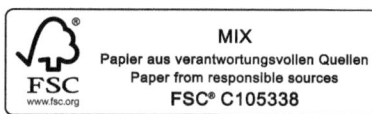

MIX
Papier aus verantwortungsvollen Quellen
Paper from responsible sources
FSC® C105338
FSC
www.fsc.org

When we think we can control any disease by vaccination,
in the foreseeable future, we dumb our immune system so
that it will no longer be able to cure the tiniest infection.
That will please the pharmaceutical industry.

I think Hippocrates, the father of modern medicine, would agree
since he demanded that our food should be our remedies.
Have you ever seen syringes hang on trees or shoot out of the ground?

I also refer to Hippocrates when choosing the title picture.
It shows fresh, fermented or pickled food.
A reader recently praised the German edition of this book,
but she also wrote: "I was repelled by the sight of the bloody fish
on the cover, although we also eat fish sometimes."

I'm always happy about feedback, especially when I can clear up
ambiguities or errors. The enzymatically matured matjes herring
on the cover is by no means bloody. My friend had brought me
some very young, not yet sexually mature herring fresh from Holland.
And these damsel herrings are silver on one side and pink on the other.

The Japanese also eat fish with rice, even raw, like sushi.
And as is well known, the Japanese life expectancy
is particularly long despite the two nuclear bombs.
The world's oldest person, Kane Tanaka, recently died at age 109.

But it's good that my readers have their say, so I can draw attention
to the importance of eating raw, fresh and unprocessed foods,
including uncooked and pickled fish.
Because heating our food above 42° C destroys the enzymes
that break down food components, lipases (fat), amylases (carbohydrates)
and proteases (protein). With raw food, you relieve your pancreas,
which can only produce a certain amount of enzymes in life.

TABLE OF CONTENTS

Don't be surprised that I back up my statements based on my studies and reports from relatives, friends, and acquaintances with so many independent studies. One proves, e. g., that 44 years ago, hydrogen peroxide (H_2O_2) inactivated the *novel* coronavirus at a concentration of 3%.

As you find out in the book, many other researchers
around the world have also tested antiviral, mostly
natural substances in test tubes and on living organisms.

And loosely based on Goethe, one of our most important poets and naturalists:
We have to repeat Truth constantly because Error is also preached
all the time and not just by a few, but by the multitude.

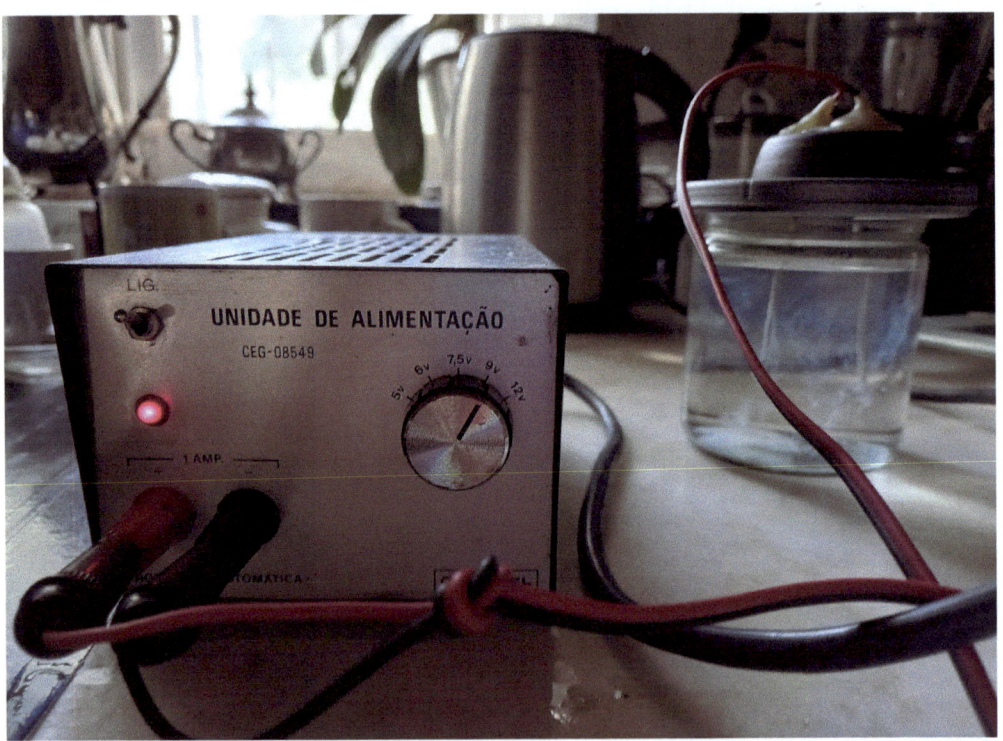

Preface

As the author of the self-help healing book "Stärke dein Immunsystem und heile dich selbst" (boost your immune system and heal yourself), you can expect that I will inform you about mobilizing your body's defenses. Perhaps, through my healthy cuisine and anti-anxiety management, I can encourage you also to trust in life and limb and achieve a less fearful relationship with death.

The motivation to dedicate me to the immune system bases on my medical history. Immunized from head to toe against childhood diseases, epidemics, and other frightening ailments, I still got all teething problems apart from polio. As a baby, I got penicillin for pneumonia. At the age of five, I had already had two operations behind me. Freed from the tonsils and appendix - two organs of the immune system - one infection followed the other. Since fought with heavy artillery, I suffered from digestive problems since antibiotics, as now well-known, destroy the healthy intestinal flora.

The parasitic yeast candida albicans took over and robbed my cells of the essential nutrients. At the age of 10, the lenses of my eyes began to cloud over. When I was 13, I had operations on the "old age star". After a series of cataract and postcataract surgeries I started an apprenticeship as a medical assistant. Probably unconsciously to learn something about the background of my ailing health. However, in the doctor's office I learned to maintain the toxin level in my body: I smoked in the waiting room after the rush of patients was over and stocked up on free appetite suppressants and dehydration pills, which the representatives of the pharmaceutical industry were not stingy. The chemical broth simmering in me resulted in hay fever of the worst kind I the first year of my adulthood, which I tried to suppress with antihistamines for lack of better knowledge.

In retrospect, it doesn't seem so strange that after a few years of work, I switched to psychology, among other things, through the second educational path. Because at the beginning of the 1970s, the search for the causes of psychosomatic illnesses was en vogue and this topic was much discussed. But even then, I did not find a solution to the riddle.

It wasn't until I began to study nutrition in the United States that I realized what most of us get sick of, namely malnutrition and an unhealthy lifestyle. Most adults now suffer from any form of allergy or degenerative disease or are completely over-acidic.

During my studies, Halima Neumann visited me in Los Angeles. The health expert found her vocation after curing herself of severe cancer with spirulina, papaya, aloe vera and wheatgrass. She familiarized me with the blue-green microalgae, which regenerate cells and are rich in vital substances. Spirulina has already recommended as a meat substitute by the West Hollywood AIDS Support Group, which I volunteered. Through Halima's suggestion I came up with the plan of doing an empirical study for my dissertation with the 300 or so young men who met every Wednesday in West Hollywood. Especially since Gustafson and colleagues discovered that the sulfonic components of the glycolipids in spirulina destroy HIV (1989).

So you will not be surprised if I would like to explain to you that you can use natural antiviral remedies as a preventative measure or in the case of the onset of viral respiratory diseases. And quickly. If, e. g., I come from a supermarket in corona times and start coughing – though the subconscious can play a trick on me – I immediately take a few drops of H_2O_2 or colloidal silver (see page 22 ff.) and some spirulina pellets. And the cough is gone. With these side effect-free remedies, you quasi install a second immune system. It is best not to give a virus that may have nested within you time or space to multiply mercilessly. Because if you don't do anything about an established virus, preventing or slowing the growth of the virus depends first and foremost on how strong your immune system is. An intact immune system will recognize the virus and fight it off before it has a chance to enter your cells. Once it enters your cells, it may be able to identify and stop the virus. This work undertake special immune cells, such as the large phagocytes (macrophages), killer cells, T cells, B cells, etc.

If your immune system is overly weak, it may not be able to do either. As a result, the virus can spread quickly and unabated and cause damage. Even medical intervention may not be enough to protect you from organ failure. Because of this, you need a strong body's defense system. To be strong, you need nutrients from food to build immune cells. If you eat a low-nutrient diet, it may not function optimally. The spirulina alga is the most nutritious food, a cornucopia of micro-nutrients that your immune system needs, including antiviral substances (see page 25 ff.).

In case you are wondering what the topic of beauty is about in this book: It's cause I became aware of a study result: 87% of the participants grew hair again six weeks after daily application of onion juice. Since tufts of hair can go out of stress, I thought that this information might be of interest to you in stressful times of pandemic measures. But since I didn't want to do the procedure a second time and found a recipe for a more pleasant application (see page 41), I skipped the onion cure in the book. You can test them yourself by going online:

https://www.instyle.de/beauty/vollere-haare-mit-zwiebelsaft

In addition to this impulse, years ago, I interviewed holistic beauticians in German-speaking countries for a book project initiated by Bob Hartmann, head of *Deynique* and *Cosmetic World*. I learned about wellness, body alignment, deacidification, pain/skin treatments, and facial muscle strengthening. And I thought it could be worth it in unruly times to manage health and beauty matters yourself. Especially when quarantine is mandatory or if beauty and hairdressing salons remain closed. It would also be a shame if the valuable tips of the experienced beauty carers lay idle. In addition, the recipe section of the book shows you super healthy dishes beneficial to your figure.

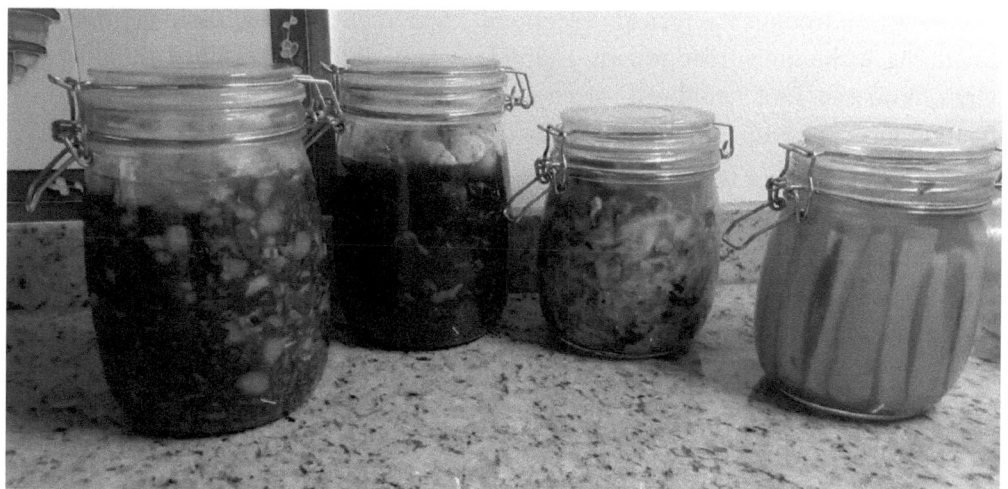

Introduction

In I. part, this new self-help healing book for perfect immune protection informs you about the reasons for our currently weakening immune system. You will also find out what you can do to support your body's defense. There is also a list of symptoms due to immune suppression.

Part II shows how you can specifically strengthen your immune system, starting with base-forming foods and lifestyles. You will also learn about the emergence and spread of human coronaviruses with analogous diseases. You can also find out about drugs tested against COVID-19 and five drugs that were said to be available in fall 2021.

Part III tells you about medicinal mushrooms and other plants, e. g. how their leaves, roots, berries, or kernels can help you regenerate and rejuvenate. Some of them have already been used successfully against SARS-CoV-2 viruses.

Part V tells you about detoxifying the body with the best foods to eliminate accumulated pollutants and avoid acidosis.

Part VI shows how scalar wave analysis quickly determines your vital substance status without lengthy and expensive laboratory tests. You can also have all bodily functions and burden with harmful substances tested promptly.

Part VII introduces physical, emotional, and mental strengthening practices, breathing techniques, recognizing individual fear, and other trained thought patterns. You can find happiness, strengthen your immune system by singing, use healing thoughts and commemorate the dead as a source of strength.

Part VIII is about delaying the aging process and training your autodidactic know-how so that your skin, hair, muscles, and tissues stay in shape even in times of crisis.

And last but not least, Part IX shows you how quickly and easily you can use the recipes from Dr Meyer's healthy cooking.

I. THE MIRACLE OF THE BODY DEFENSE

If your immune system is intact, it protects you from germs and environmental toxins. The healthy intestinal flora makes a significant contribution to the functioning of your immune system. Our intestinal bacteria not only help with the utilization of food components. If we, e. g., eat something rotten, they also prevent pathogens from spreading. Therefore, a healthy microbiome is a basis for an intact immune system.

If we have a cold, our immune system fights against unwanted pathogens. And the germs are in for it now so that bacteria, viruses, and parasites are just harmless little guys. Since our body is full of toxins and once again confronted with them, the immune system detects and neutralizes pollutants from food and the environment and eliminates most of them. It also succeeds in the fight against cancer cells, which we contract now and then, e. g. in case of nutritional errors, in shock situations, or when we are under permanent stress.

Reasons for a generally weakening immune system

People have tried to adapt to chemical substances in food and the environment for the past seventy years. However, according to its genetic makeup, our body depends on gently prepared foods that have matured in light, clean air, and sun. But our food today consists mainly of "dead matter".

The fossil of a 5 feet tall, upright pre-hominid found in Ethiopia suggests that human-like predecessors ate freshly harvested plants and unpolluted meat and fish for more than four million years. Their days were full of hard physical labor, most of which might have been gathering food and protection against wild animals.

Therefore, it is impossible to assume that we can adapt to denatured food in a tiny fraction of this time without harming our body, mind, and spirit.

In memory of Hippocrates, the father of modern medicine, we can today change his apt statement concerning health-promoting or health-maintaining vegetable foods as following headline postulates:

Let biodynamically grown food be our medicine

Let's see how radical our diet has changed over the past hundred years. Instead of the earlier crop rotation cultivation, in which the arable land lies fallow for a year after six years, the conventional production is over-exploiting Mother Earth. The farmers fog their fields with toxic substances and remove the nutrient-rich outer shell of the grain, which anyway grows on depleted soils.

People with a weak immune system would be better off reducing the amount of food they eat anyhow because then there would be less digestive work, fewer toxin s would enter the body, and thus our immune cells would have less work. That is especially true in cases of acute illness. But when I say that, I usually run into a wall and keep hearing: But you have to eat!

No, you don't have to! We always heal faster if we eat as little as possible and drink a lot of pure water, cause then the body's defense has less trouble with the toxins in the food and our intestinal bacteria have less work.

The animals show us how they behave when they are not well: they eat grass and drink water. We can also grow barley grass in a litter box, chew the juice from the stalks and drink water with it. But it is easier with spirulina fasting. After all, the precursors of these blue-green microalgae are the first descendants of the first photosynthetic life form and created our oxygen atmosphere about three and a half billion years ago. With the help of sunlight, they were able to split water molecules, thereby generating their food from the surrounding gases and minerals. The blue-green algae transformed the earth into a life-friendly system and created the conditions for the development of multicellular organisms. We can therefore call them the parent substance of flora and fauna. And all of the vital substances we need for life can be obtained from this blue-green micro-alga, or more precisely from the cyanobacteria.

Children are at great risk from heavy metals and pesticides

The little ones are particularly sensitive to pesticides, as their rapidly growing cells are more susceptible to carcinogens than the cells of adults. Children also inhale higher doses of toxins for their body weight than adults and tend to breathe through their mouths rather than through their noses. This eliminates the filter function of

14

the nasal cilia. And finally, their small size causes increased absorption of toxins. Because small children are closer to the exhaust pipes of the vehicles and are more likely to come into contact with the pesticides on the lawn or fields through playing and romping around.

Lack of exercise and sleep weaken the immune system

Today's predominantly sedentary professional activity and the lack of movement in leisure time have a particularly detrimental effect on the metabolism and the cardio-vascular system. Especially when we only sit in front of the TV or surf the Internet in our free time.

We weren't born with engines. We can therefore assume creation intended that we move our bodies vigorously. Today we no longer have to chase after our food, rub the laundry and drag the water into the house. Because of the relief that our modern way of life has brought, we hardly see ourselves having to make any effort. There-fore, it is highly advisable to keep fit with leisure activities. Otherwise, we become obese, depressed, tense, and angry.

We also get angry and irritable when we sleep little. Sleeping teas or pills are less good solutions. It is better to determine the cause, such as late dinners or taking medication. Consuming of too much alcohol, caffeine, drugs, legumes, hard cheese, meat, fat, protein-rich and spicy foods, fast food, sweets, leafy salads, and raw veg-etables can disturb your sleep also. Perhaps there is a shortage of melatonin, vitamin B3, vitamin C, magnesium, or copper. Or the eternal salad of thoughts plagues. It is often helpful to inhale deeply several times, tensing all muscles and letting them go when you exhale. The jingling of your eyelashes also makes you tired, and you can fall asleep more quickly. That brings us to another reason for sleep disorders: lack of movement.

Radiation exposure puts a strain on the immune system

We are surrounded by ionizing radiation, which depends on its strength and duration, restricts cellular function or can lead to cell death. Even moderate exposure to x-rays, electrosmog from computers, televisions, microwave ovens and other devices can lead to headaches, nausea, vomiting, poor appetite and diarrhea.

Long-term radiation exposure can result in sterility, deformities, leukemia or other forms of cancer, hair loss and cataracts. The radiation we expose ourselves to during an intercontinental flight is roughly equivalent to three x-ray images of the lungs. Radiation doses too low to destroy cells can still cause cellular changes that, years later, suppress the immune system or cause thyroid problems.

Other factors that negatively affect the immune system

We recognize a weakening immune system by having colds, coughs, sore throats or other cold symptoms often or longer and stronger than usual. It happens mainly when our body is more susceptible to illnesses, i. e. under stress, grief and hormonal changes. Furthermore, feelings of hatred, resentment, envy, suppressed worries, and a lack of zest for life can weaken our body's defenses.

Intoxicants or stimulants give the immune system wrong signals, so that it reacts irritated and misdirected. Since it is capable of learning, there is a risk that it will behave incorrectly again in the future in response to similar stimulation.

Psychological stress, nervousness and anxiety in everyday situations, i. e., during work, in traffic or at home, also influence the immune system negatively.

If we eat a lot and consume too much fat or sugar, the immune system has to send defense cells into the digestive tract. These must remove from possible sources of inflammation. There is, therefore, a risk of infection.

Symptoms that may be due to immune suppression

If you discover any signs of immune suppression listed below in yourself or a loved one, you better take immediate action to strengthen your body's defenses.

Acne that persists beyond the hormonal cycle of puberty, which completes by the age of 25.

Allergies are a false reaction of the immune system. Dangerous immune complexes flood organism, and removing them is an enormous burden.

Coated tongue that lasts for more than three weeks.

Middle-aged high blood pressure is a sign of narrowed, inflexible veins due to arteriosclerosis due to deposited immune complexes.

Type II diabetes (outbreak in adulthood) shows that enzyme production in the pancreas - crucial for the perfect functioning of the immune system - has decreased.

Colds, more than two to three times a year, or any cold that lasts more than three weeks

Flu, more than once a year

Skin that becomes dry and wrinkled after age 30 to 35 is a sign that the production of sex hormones is decreasing. In a healthy body, all hormones are in balance.

Herpes infections indicate a not properly working immune system, although that does not mean one is susceptible to other infections.

Tonsillitis, more than once a year

Stiff limbs n the morning can be an onset of rheumatic disease, also related to an irritated immune system.

Warts, which occur particularly frequently during puberty, pregnancy and menopause, indicate a tolerated viral infection and are sign of a weakened immune system.

Dental infections or wound-healing that takes more than three weeks

When and how are we more susceptible to disease?

In hormonal changes, puberty, pregnancy or menopause, we are particularly prone to health problems.

But there is also an increased risk of illness during periods of mourning, shock or extreme fear.

Constant stress and unfavorable environmental factors, including lockdown measures associated with the coronavirus, can also lead to physical and mental illnesses.

And last but not least, food poisons, fast food and today's convenience food culture are further factors that make our bodies more susceptible to diseases.

II. IMMUNE BOOSTER AND HELP WITH CORONA

Strengthen your immune system with a diet rich in vital substances, pure water, sunlight, lots of exercise in the fresh air and enough sleep. Then you can trust your inner healer to the point that it will protect you from serious illness even in times of mass illnesses.

COVID-19: the infectious disease caused by the coronavirus

Several human coronaviruses (HCoVs) seem capable of creating epidemics or pandemics. The correlating diseases characterized by severe respiratory disease, such as Severe Acute Respiratory Syndrome (SARS-CoV), the Middle East CoV and today SARS-CoV-2, broke out uncontrollably in December 2019 and around the world supposedly killed five million people. The first incidence of COVID-19 happened in Hubei, Wuhan, China, in late December 2019. Since the borders of the affected region were not closed in time, COVID-19 spread like wildfire through air travel almost all over the world. The viral lower respiratory-tract-infection thought to be caused by zoonotic diseases. That means when pathogens jump from animals to humans, as some suspect, from bats. Others think they know it was a laboratory accident.

How does COVID-19 attack your respiratory system or other organ systems? It infects and inflames your lungs, which thus cannot take in enough oxygen or remove carbon dioxide. It is ultimately so damaged that it fails. The virus appears to toss out the iron atom in your hemoglobin and replace it with itself. First, the iron atom in your hemoglobin carries oxygen into your blood. Is it removed and replaced by the virus, your hemoglobin can no longer carry oxygen into your body, possibly leading to organ failure. Many COVID-19 patients die of cardiac arrest because their heart does not get enough oxygen.

Due to the high number of deaths, economic losses and impairments, further examination is needed to what extent existing alternatives can mitigate the progress of the pandemic or kill the virus.

As I said before, there is always something you can do to help a mild course of a viral disease: Eat fresh food, drink pure water, sleep 7–8 hours, and exercise a lot in the fresh air. Thus you have already laid the foundation for a stable immune system.

However, since you no longer get enough vital substances from food due to depleted arable land, you better identify your deficiencies and compensate for them with appropriate food supplements. See page 56 ff.

Below you will find evidence that you can protect yourself with certain medicinal substances, but above all with natural food supplements, as if by a second immune system.

Are mRNA vaccines worse than the disease?

The US government-initiated public-private partnership, Operation Warp Speed, launched two mRNA vaccines in the United States, manufactured by Pfizer and Moderna. The interim results promised high efficacy for both vaccines. It helped substantiate the FDA's emergency approval with arguments. However, the extremely rapid spread of these vaccines through controlled trials and mass adoption raises several safety concerns.

The inoculated lipid nanoparticles in the BioNTech vaccine contain cationic peptides. These were known as highly toxic and DNA-destructive for many years! The cell biologist Dr Vanessa Schmidt-Krüger explains that cationic peptides damage liver cells and make them inoperable. The vaccinated person can only survive by eliminating the cationic lipids, which is barely attainable with previous illnesses. The vaccinated person has to enable the body to intercept oxygen radicals. Among the most potent free radical scavengers are apigenin, arginine, astaxanthin, organic acerola, cranberry, glutathione, lupine proteins, melatonin, NAC, methylene blue, quercetin, rice/pea proteins, terpenes, and their blending. By the way, glutathione is supposed to prevent the spike protein from docking on the ACE2 receptor. The functions of the other radical scavengers you will find under the following link:

http://www.borderlands.de/Links/Edinger821BewusstTV.pdf

US researchers Stephanie Seneff (Computer Science and Artificial Intelligence Laboratory, MIT, Cambridge) and Greg Nigh (Naturopathic Oncology, Immersion Health, Portland, OR) reviewed possible unintended consequences of mRNA vaccines against COVID-19. They found the innate immune suppression by SARS-CoV-2 mRNA vaccinations. They also induce a variety of pathologies such as blood diseases, neurodegenerative diseases and autoimmune diseases. Under these possibly unleashed pathologies, the authors discussed the relevance of animal protein-related

amino acid sequences within the spike protein. They also presented a brief overview of studies showing the potential for *spike protein shedding*, the transmission of the protein from a vaccinated to an unvaccinated person. This leads to symptoms produced in the latter. Finally, they addressed a common point of discussion, namely whether or not these vaccines could alter the DNA of the vaccinated people. While there are no studies to prove this, they presented a plausible scenario supported by previously established pathways for converting and transporting genetic material, according to which injected mRNA could ultimately incorporate into germ cell DNA for transgenerational delivery. Finally, the authors recommend surveillance, which will help to clarify the long-term effects of these experimental drugs and to assess the risk-benefit ratio of these novel technologies
https://www.ncbi.nlm.nih.gov/pmc/articles/PMC8720447/

On June 28th, 2021, the Madrid professor Dr Pablo Campra observed via optical and electronic microscopy graphene oxide in aqueous suspension (ComirnatyTM) (RD1) in the mRNA vaccines from Pfizer and Moderna.
https://www.researchgate.net/publication/354059739
https://www.europarl.europa.eu/doceo/document/P-9-2022-000303_EN.html

Guangbo Qu and his ten Beijing collegues were able to show in their study that graphene oxide (GO) triggered necrotic cell death in macrophages. GO exposure also caused a massive increase in intracellular reactive oxygen species (ROS), which contributed to the cause of cell death. Cytoskeletal damage and oxidative stress also led to reduced viability and function of large phagocytes during GO treatment. Qu et al., ACS nano. 2013 Jul 23; 7 (7): 5732-45

**In many different Chinese, Korean and other patent applications,
graphene is included as a component of covid-vaccines.
Graphene is a toxic material for the human body.**

That explains dozens of scientific papers and should therefore not included in vaccines.

Promising agents against SARS-CoV-2 and mutants

Chloroquine is supposedly not recommended to treat COVID-19. Why not? What do you think? My guess: too cheap. Martin J. Vincent and his American colleagues stated already in 2005 that Chloroquine, a relatively safe, effective and inexpensive drug used for treating, e. g., malaria, amoebiosis and *HIV*, inhibits the infection and spread of SARS-CoV in cell culture!

At the end of June 2021, the European Commission on the development and availability of COVID-19 therapeutics published five treatment candidates that may be available for treating patients across the EU.

"The five products are at an advanced stage of development and have high potential to be among the three new COVID-19 therapeutics that will receive approval by October 2021, provided the final data demonstrate their safety, quality and effectiveness. The products are:

New COVID-19 indications for existing drugs:

Baricitinib by Eli Lilly

Newly developed monoclonal antibodies:

Combination of Bamlanivimab and Etesevimab by Eli Lilly

Combination of casirivimab and imdevimab from Regeneron Pharmaceuticals, Inc. and F. Hoffman-La Roche, Ltd.

Regdanivimab from Celltrion

Sotrovimab from GlaxoSmithKline and Vir Biotechnology, Inc. "

https://ec.europa.eu/germany/news/20210629-coronavirus-therapeutika_de

This EU strategy does not strike me as glorious as shown. Especially since, as I show in the book, there are already numerous therapeutic agents. And consider that in Butane, Thailand and China there were only 1 to 3 corona deaths per million inhabitants, but in Germany more than 800. Because while in Germany, every patient goes to the doctor an average of 17 times a year, whereas the people in aforenamed countries only see doctors if they have symptoms. I do not even then, but fast and take H_2O_2, colloidal silver & Co. Probably five years ago, I already suffered from a COVID-19 infection. I coughed for months and had no sense of smell for over a year. But so far, I have not needed an antibody test. And my loyal readers know that I avoid medical practices.

21

In their study, the US researchers Martin D. Hellwig and Anabela Maia also drew attention to the fact that Ivermectin, a drug for the treatment of parasitic worms, is receiving a lot of attention worldwide as an effective agent against COVID-19 (2021).

The idea of also using the preparation to treat coronaviruses came from Latin America, where doctors in some countries used it successfully. More recently, studies have suggested this treatment might be effective, but more research would be needed. I would advise my readers to do their research if they suspect acute respiratory syndrome. Then:

Only if you can stand up to viruses quickly,
you have the best chance for a mild course.

Carlos KH Wong, Eric YF Wan and their twelve Hong Kong and Chinese research colleagues examined various options for treating COVID-19 in two Chinese case cohorts, one in Hong Kong SAR and one in Anhui, China. They analyzed 4,771 symptomatic patients from Hong Kong between January 21 and December 6, 2020, and 648 symptomatic patients from Anhui between January 1 and February 27, 2020. In doing so, they censored all observations as of December 13, 2020, from the time from hospital admission to discharge and all therapeutic options. They looked at lopinavir-ritonavir, ribavirin, umifenovir, interferon-alpha-2b, interferon-beta-1b, corticosteroids, antibiotics, and Chinese medicines. And also four interferon-beta-1b combination treatment groups.

The study results advocate early administration
of interferon-beta-1b alone or in combination with
oral ribavirin in COVID-19 patients!

Following, you will find my choice of treatments for all kinds of viruses, including corona..

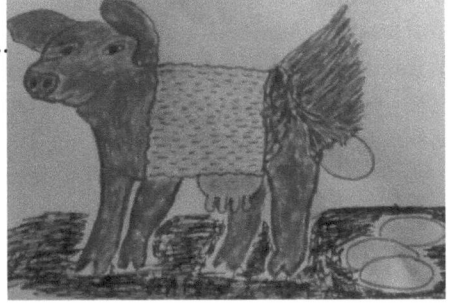

H2O2: an all-rounder called the egg-laying woolly milk sow of medicine

Hydrogen peroxide is an ordinary and versatile medicinal agent used for more than a hundred years against fungi, bacteria and viruses. For it destroys the lipid layer of viruses and can inactivate microbes. When so by destroying the envelope, the viruses become harmless H_2O_2 can also help against the coronaviruses.

While searching for COVID-19 or SARS-CoV data, I discovered an exciting study performed almost half a century ago! Mentel and his Russian research colleagues did not treat the coronavirus as anything special. However, while searching for this researcher, I came across human abysses: multiple defenestrations from people who had to do with COVID-19. But in the land of the "flawless democrat" (Gerhard Schröder), people are less squeamish about human life.
aerztezeitung.de/Nachrichten/Russischer-Corona-Forscher-nach-Fenster-sturz-gestorben-415815

The effect of H_2O_2 on adenovirus types 3 and 6, adenovirus type 4, rhinoviruses 1A, 1B and type 7, myxoviruses, influenza A and B, respiratory syncytial virus, strain Long and coronavirus strain 229E was tested in vitro with various H_2O_2-concentration and exposure time investigated.

H_2O_2 at a concentration of 3 per cent inactivated all of them examined viruses within 1 to 30 minutes. Coronaviruses and influenza viruses proved to be the most sensitive.

Retroviruses, adenoviruses and adeno-associated viruses were relatively stable. (1977) H_2O_2 is a particularly simple means of virus inactivation. But first I always try colloidal silver because it is tasteless and when applied externally, unlike H_2O_2 or iodine, it doesn't burn.

H_2O_2 is unrivaled cheap, cannot be patented, is available in pharmacies and online shops without a prescription and has no resistance whatsoever. Therefore, the pharmaceutical industry may not be amused that I dust it off again. For more than 100 years, the remedy has been recognized, and countless studies have proven its effectiveness against a wide variety of diseases, even the dreaded lung cancer.

In a test tube test, hydrogen peroxide inhibited the growth of Calu-6 and A549 lung cancer cells through cell death and G1 phase arrest.

(Park WH 2018)

The oxygen water is more than two hundred years old. Because: In 1818, the French chemist Louis Jacques Thenard (1777-1857) treated a barium salt, which the famous

Alexander von Humboldt (1769-1859) had first produced in Paris in 1799, with strong acids (such as sulfuric acid) and obtained a dilute, substance dissolved in water. The chemist was astonished that it disintegrated when adding traces of metal, blood or bases, forming oxygen and leaving only water. The substance was initially called "oxygenated water" (Gartz 2014). Jochen Gartz uses the proven but forgotten home remedy that kills antibiotic-resistant germs. Namely, 8 to 25 drops of 35% food-grade hydrogen peroxide dissolved in 240 ml of water or aloe juice three times a day. Currently, you can buy only up to 9 %. You can start with 20 drops and work up to 60 or from a teaspoon to a tablespoon full.

Personal experience: Years ago, I was able to remove an ulcer in my husband's neck with H2O2. I brushed it with a cotton swab 2-3 times a day until it broke open after a few weeks and a green, foul-smelling liquor came out.

I recommended a friend with gum problems to treat the area with a cotton swab dipped in H2O2. Karl, who was already a little bit fussy at the time, literally came to life. Because he found that hydrogen peroxide was also suitable for many other of his ailments.

I take it myself when I feel uncomfortable in the gastrointestinal area, when I discover a pimple or suspicious spot or for wound treatment. But also when unwanted microorganisms get out of hand in my body.

Colloidal silver: universal antibiotic for humans and animals

For years I've been making CS, a broad-spectrum antibiotic with no side effects using 99.9% silver rods. At first, only with a 9-volt battery and contact cables, now as shown on page 8. With the plastic lid, the rods fit into almost any glass. The odorless and tasteless silver water has been used against viruses, bacteria, fungi and parasites for around a hundred years. If you eat with silver cutlery, there is a good chance that the microbes will find another host instead of you.

Allegedly there are no effective antiviral measures against COVID-19. Silver nanoparticles (AgNP) have antiviral properties and are supposed to inhibit SARS-CoV-2. Due to the need for an effective agent against SARS-CoV-2, Sundararaj S. Jeremiah and his colleagues investigated the antiviral effects of AgNPs. They tested a variety of silver nanoparticles of different sizes and concentrations, finding that particles with a diameter of about 10 nm at concentrations between 1 and 10 ppm were effective in inhibiting extracellular SARS-CoV-2! (Jeremiah et al. 2020)

The cranberry has the potential to kill the SARS-CoV-2 virus

Cranberries have long been valued for their nutritional and medicinal properties. They are used to relieve stomach ailments, liver problems and bowel disorders. Today, cranberry products are most frequently used to help the body manage symptoms of Urinary Tract Infections. (Meyer 2017)

Cranberry contains proanthocyanidins, also known as proanthocyanidins or condensed tannins. They make it impossible for microorganisms to adhere to the growth of the human body, thus reducing the probability of acquired infections. They improve atherosclerosis, restore elasticity, prevent multiple arterial blood flow from cardiovascular disease, and significantly improve outcomes. Cranberry's vitamin C, iron, antioxidants, and proanthocyanidins are abundant to prevent cell damage while maintaining cell health and vitality, leaving skin soft and rosy.

As early as 2005, E.I. Weiss and his colleagues found that cranberry juice components affect the adherence and infectivity of the influenza virus.

Roberta Giordo and her research colleagues show that Cranberries' resveratrol is a promising supplement to prevent and treat COVID-19. (2021)

Spirulina, a fountain of youth and candidate against corona & co

Spirulina platensis is probably the most globally researched food supplement. Animal breeders knew the *blue-green miracle*, which not only regenerates and balances the human body and mind, even before I made it known in German-speaking and Eastern European countries. Because the micro-alga, which is unparalleled in terms of vital substances, has long been an insider tip for happy and healthy, high performance horses and brightly colored lively fish and birds. Meanwhile also athletes around the globe use spirulina for its energizing, mood lifting, pain relieving and muscle tissue repairing effect of.

If you want to stay healthy, strengthening your immunity is the easiest way for your body to resist viral infection. In this context, spirulina, the survival food for a new age (M. Meyer 2016), seems to be a potential panacea. Because the microalga was able to clinically strengthen immunity against viral diseases several times. In addition to an abundance of vitamins and minerals, it contains C-phycocyanin, a pigment-binding protein that strengthens the antioxidant, inflammatory and anti-tumor effects. Anti-flu efficacy studies showed that a spirulina extract inhibited viral plaque formation in a variety of influenza viruses, including oseltamivir-resistant strains. (Chen et al., 2016)

The high versatility of viruses has hindered the development of vaccines. Strains resistant to existing antiviral drugs have also emerged. Therefore, side-effect-free food supplements are becoming more and more crucial. Spirulina extracts have diverse therapeutic effects, including lowering cholesterol, immune modulation, antioxidant, anticancer and antiviral effects. (Meyer 2016)

Particularly benefiting from spirulina are the sick, convalescent, heavy workers, athletes, stressed mothers, hyperactive children, the elderly and busy managers.

The Maya and Aztecs of ancient Central America already appreciated the strengthening and regenerating effects of the algae and used them daily in their food. They used baskets to scoop the green foam from the shallow Lake Chad. Some researchers believe that the lichen crusting on rocks and soil is the manna mentioned in the Bible. God is said to have given this symbiosis of fungus and blue-green algae to the starving Israelis in the desert. The story provides two dozen more concrete examples of this source of protein and vital substances used in soups, sauces or as a spread.

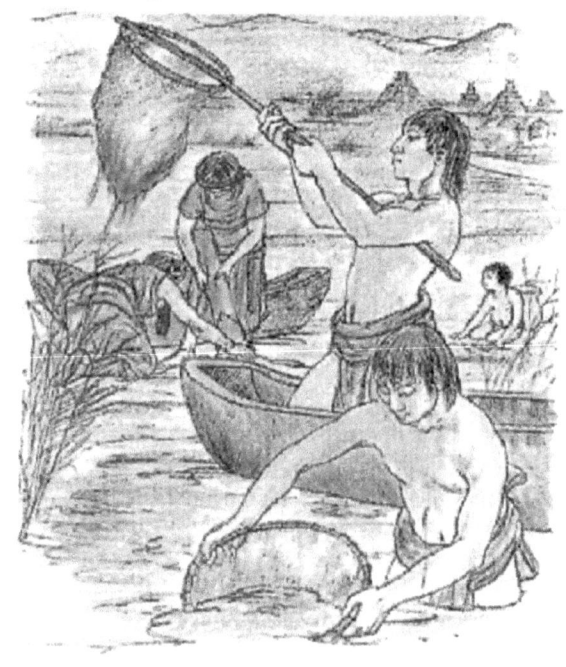

But it was not until 1940 that the phycologist Pierre-Augustin Dangeard and 1964 the botanist Jean Leonhard reported on the customs of the Kanembu people: They scooped the strange blue-green foam from the surface of Lake Chad and allowed it to dry into cakes. In 1967 Hiroshi Nakamura became aware of the spirulina projects run by the French National Petroleum Center. He had been interested in algae as a source of protein for the starving world for a long time and was enthusiastic about the variety of uses of this high-quality species.

Spirulinas's peptides, phycobiliproteins, sulphated polysaccharides, and calcium spirulan suggests spirulina's potential role in warding off infection and the progression of COVID-19 disease. (Ratha et al., 2021)

Giselle Pentón-Rol and her Cuban and Californian colleagues who study longevity, genetic engineering, and biological assessments provide an overview of recent research on spirulina. In one study, rodents got C-phycocyanin, a pigment-protein complex from spirulina. It showed protective effects in ischemic stroke and multiple sclerosis. The authors, therefore, suggest that spirulina's active ingredients also have a protective effect against Alzheimer's and Parkinson's disease, as well as COVID-19 and its neurological complications. (Pentón-Rol et al., 2021)

As I said before, the virus appears to be throwing out the iron atom in hemoglobin and replacing it with itself. And since the iron atom in hemoglobin transports oxygen into the blood, the hemoglobin can no longer transport oxygen into the body, what can lead to acute respiratory distress syndrome and organ failure. Many COVID-19 patients die of cardiac arrest because their hearts deprived of oxygen.

Asaf Tzachor and his Israeli and Icelandic research colleagues found an extract of photosynthetically enhanced spirulina to reduce the immune system's release of a protein by 70 percent. It can trigger a cytokine storm in the lungs, leading to acute respiratory distress and organ damage.They published their study in the journal Marine Biotechnology. An extract from the microalgae, or rather the cyanobacterium *Spirulina* or *Athrospira platensis*, can help COVID-19 patients avoid serious illnesses. Therefore, according to Tzachor, it can prevent cytokine storms when given to patients soon after diagnosis. The researchers recommend timely studies in animal models and humans to determine the effectiveness of a natural, algae-based treatment for viral cytokine storms and acute respiratory distress syndrome and investigate the suitability of a novel anti-TNF-alpha therapy. (Tzachor et al., 2021)

Whether you take the pellets or the 100% pure powder is up to you. I've been using both for over thirty years. This could be the reason why I have hardly ever gray hair and have not suffered any severe illnesses during this time, though as a child, I was so brimful with anesthetics and medicines that Prof Jäger pricked my senile cataract at the age of 13. You can see my enthusiasm from the fact that I have already written seven books on the beneficial microalgae for people of all ages and animals: all with delicious recipes and exciting information.

Personal experience: When I feel down after a thought, I realize that I realize that I have not used spirulina in a while. The same applies when my eyes itch. A few minutes after sucking some pallets or drinking a spirulina smoothy, my mood improves, or my allergic reactions disappear.

My father had to take two insulin tablets for his diabetes. After taking one spirulina tablet morning, noon and night for a while, he only needed 1/2 insulin tablet. But I could not convince him to take two spirulina each time. Maybe he needed his daily finger prick.

Cannabis: potential help in the fight against corona

Cannabidiol (CBD) has gained more and more attention in recent years. Like the more well-known psychoactive "high" agent THC, CBD is an extract from the cannabis plant. Medical professionals prescribe CBD for various health problems. It could also help against corona due to its anti-inflammatory and antioxidant effects. Preclinical data show that CBD promises relief in anxiety memory processing, improved sleep, and depression, often associated with anxiety. Therefore, CBD could become a promising new treatment option for COVID-related post-traumatic stress disorder. These should be investigated and tested in appropriately designed randomized controlled studies. (Sullivan et al., 2021)

To test the effect of CBD on SARS-CoV-2 replication, Long Chi Nguyen and her US research colleagues pretreated human A549 lung cancer cells with 0-10 µM CBD for two hours before infection with SARS-CoV. After 48 hours, they monitored the cells for the expression of the viral spike protein. For comparison, they treated about the same number of cells with the mixed lineage kinase inhibitor URMC-099, which they previously used as an antiviral against HIV, and with other inhibitors. All three inhibitors blocked virus replication. CBD also inhibited SARS-CoV-2 replication in kidney epithelial cells. These results show:

CBD can block SARS-CoV-2 infection in its early stages and when you use it, you have a lower risk of SARS-CoV-2-infection.

CBD was also able to inhibit the replication of mouse hepatitis virus (MHV). Since the researchers did not observe toxicity at the effective
 doses, there is a possibility that CBD could be effective against new pathogenic viruses emerging in the future. (Nguyen 2021)

Users report success with headaches, depression and tension. I had good experiences with CBD oil for inflammatory pain in the wrists and for sleep disorders.

Vitamin D affects the risk of death from COVID 19

Up until now, we believed that low vitamin D levels only risked osteoporosis and rickets. However, a study shows that certain underlying diseases such as diabetes, cardiovascular diseases, being very overweight and high blood pressure increase the risk of a severe course if a COVID-19 infection occurs. These diseases and autoimmune diseases, depression, dementia and chronic pain are associated with low vitamin D levels. That also applies to older people, in whom a vitamin D deficiency is common and are among the risk groups. The nutritionist Prof Dr Hans-Konrad Biesalski from the University of Hohenheim in Stuttgart, evaluated 30 studies and discovered a vitamin D deficit as a possible indicator of the severity and mortality rate of COVID-19 disease. The Cochrane meta-analysis from more than 56 randomized studies totalling 95,286 participants showed: A good vitamin D supply significantly reduces the general mortality in older people, regardless of whether they live independently or are residents.

https://clinicaltrials.gov/ct2/results?cond=vitamin+D+and+Covid-19
https://www.presseportal.de/pm/113214/4871249

The vitamin D supply could also play a role during the disease because the sun vitamin regulates the immune system and the inflammatory processes in the body. How are vitamin D and the coronavirus related? As a hormone, vitamin D fulfils many different functions in the body: It ensures stout bones. It makes a decisive contribution to the normal working of the muscles and the immune system and guarantees the production of antibodies (T cells), thus curbing inflammation. These factors can notably affect infections. Therefore, Biesalski recommends keeping an eye on vitamin D levels in the event of COVID-19, especially in people who are over 65 years old and those who are seldom outdoors.

The formation in the skin from sunlight is the most important source of vitamin D. But, this only works to a limited extent in old age. In addition to the immune system, vitamin D also regulates the so-called renin-angiotensin system (RAS), which is particularly important for regulating blood pressure. In the case of an infection, vitamin D ensures that these two systems do not get out of hand. "Since the coronavirus attacks an important switching point in these control circuits, pro-inflammatory and anti-inflammatory processes are no longer in balance, Biesalski explains: "Since the coronavirus attacks an important switching point in these control circuits, pro-inflammatory and anti-inflammatory processes are no longer in balance", explains Biesalski.

The system can no longer be in control, especially if there is also a vitamin D deficiency. Then the pro-inflammatory processes pick up speed and lead to changes in the alveoli. These cause a severe complication of COVID-19 disease: acute respiratory distress syndrome (ARDS).

If a COVID-19 infection is suspected, you better check the vitamin D status and correct a possible deficit quickly, the doctor advises. Vitamin D levels are often devastatingly low in people in retirement homes. Also, when working from home, many people stay in closed rooms for long periods, contributing to a poor vitamin D supply.

However, Biesalski emphasizes that vitamin D is not a drug to cure COVID-19 diseases. But one can alleviate the course of the disease by enabling the organism to restore the balance between the pro-and anti-inflammatory processes.

A sufficient vitamin D level can hardly come about through food, according to Biesalski. Although oily fish and sun-dried mushrooms contain a lot of vitamin D. (Biesalski 2015)

Raman Kumar and his Indian research colleagues addressed the possible role of vitamin D in influencing the immune response and immunopathology associated with COVID-19. This branch of biomedical science studies the immune responses following a cytokine storm in severely affected individuals. Because most people who died in intensive care units were extremely vitamin D deficient, researchers believe this area needs serious investigation. Older people with a weak immune system and associated comorbidities are more susceptible to disturbed immune responses. Because most of them also have a severe vitamin D deficiency. As a result, vital organs in the body, including the lungs and cardiovascular system, are severely damaged. Scientists are therefore also interested in the study to assess the role of vitamin D in reducing the risk of COVID-19.

Vitamin D is a crucial regulator of the renin-angiotensin system. In addition to blood pressure, the hormone system mentioned above also regulates fluid and electrolyte balance plus systemic vascular resistance. SARS-CoV-2 uses vitamin D to enter host cells. In addition, it alters several mechanisms of the immune system, e.g., contain the virus and the replication of SARS-CoV-2, inhibit the concentration of pro-inflammatory cytokines and activate the immune cells. This article demonstrates the urgency of the evidence needed through randomized controlled trials and largely population-based ecological studies to assess the potential role of vitamin D in COVID-19. (Kumar et al., 2021)

In the meantime, I advise you to do your research,
have your vitamin D status checked, and, if necessary, take vitamin D.

However, Brit Adrian R Martineau and his numerous international research colleagues had already systematically reviewed vitamin D supplementation for preventing acute respiratory infections 4½ years ago. With due respect, one could have been a little more prepared for the cause of COVID-19, because the researchers evaluated the overall effect of vitamin D administration on the risk of an acute respiratory infection in 25 randomized controlled studies with at least 11,321 participants aged 0 to 95 years. And with the following result:

The administration of vitamin D reduced the risk of an acute respiratory infection in all participants. The scientists concluded that vitamin D supplementation was safe and chiefly protected against acute respiratory infections. Patients with a very high vitamin D deficiency could benefit most from the vitamin D supplement. (Martineau et al., 2017)

It is, therefore, better to provide your body with sufficient vitamin D at all times, especially in winter. Since COVID-19, SARS-CoV-2, and other variants are very reluctant to stay in organisms with a high vitamin D status. Therefore we can conclude that vitamin D can protect against corona.

To rule out a deficiency, you first have the vitamin D level in your blood determined. You can achieve this without taking blood via scalar waves. (Meyer 2020)

Depending on the degree of the deficiency, you can increase your exposure to the sun or use correspondingly high doses of the sun vitamin or foods containing vitamin D. Good old cod liver oil includes the most vitamin D. Also, all types of fatty fish, such as eel, kippers, herring, salmon, mackerel, avocados, eggs, mushrooms, processed cheese, Gouda and Emmental. With all the fatty, mainly acid-forming food, please don't forget the alkaline vegetables!

There are so many other natural therapeutic strategies for COVID-19 that, if applied in time, would suppress SARS-CoV-2 replication.

III. REJUVENATION AND ANTI-CORONA PLANTS FROM A TO Z

Who doesn't want to be healthy and beautiful at old age? Although we age in the course of our lives, chronological age does not always correspond to the biological age of our bodies. Our body cells and tissues change depending on our lifestyle, environmental influences and genetic predisposition. It is particularly evident in the connective tissue. The organs also change more or less quickly. We can measure age-related changes in various bio-molecules. But the pattern of epigenetic deposits also reveals the biological age.

However, you can genetically rejuvenate yourself in just a few weeks through a special diet, lots of sleep and exercise. The American Kara N. Fitzgerald and her eleven research colleagues proved this in a pilot study. The Test subjects reduced their epigenetic age by a good three years in eight weeks. They conducted a randomized controlled clinical trial on 43 healthy adult males aged 50-72 years. The eight-week treatment program included diet, sleep, exercise and relaxation recommendations, moderate intermittent fasting with lots of vegetables, little animal protein and carbohydrates, nuts, seeds, supplemental probiotics (lactic acid bacteria) and phytonutrients. The control group received no offer. Diet and lifestyle treatment were associated with a 3.23-year decrease in life compared to controls (p=0.018). The average decline in triglycerides (-25%, p=0.009) was also significant.

"This is the first evidence of a reversal of the epigenetic aging process in a randomized controlled clinical trial," state Fitzgerald and her team. It is exciting that the change in lifestyle and diet has such a profound effect on the methylation pattern of the DNA after such a short time. Indicated was this effect already in other studies, e. g., after a period of the Mediterranean diet. However, the observed changes were less clear. (Fitzgerald 2022)

In a recent study, Raphaëlle Chaix from the Sorbonne in Paris and her international research colleagues showed that long-term regular meditation could help slow down the epigenetic clock and be a prevention strategy for age-related chronic diseases. (Chaix et al., 2017)

Vaccinations and chemotherapy often appear as the only alternatives. It's also good business for the disease industry. With every vaccination, the infection increasing antibodies can form. Therefore, I am more afraid of vaccinations than of the disease.

Because I can protect myself against diseases by taking measures to strengthen the immune system, I list them in more detail on the following pages.

The amount of reports of alternatives, supported by international studies, is irrefutable evidence that foods and herbs have potential antiviral ability against SARS-CoV-2. COVID-19 infection is mainly transmitted through close contact with an infected person via respiratory droplets or touching a contaminated surface.

In the following, I will show you, among other things, medicinal plants that are effective against germs, strengthen the immune system and have a rejuvenating effect from A to Z without you having to fear undesirable side effects. Even if I repeat myself:

It was Hippocrates, the father of modern medicine, who demanded that natural food should be our remedy.

Because of the current level of knowledge, this would be, e. g., from A to Z: apricots, avocado, berries, carrots, chard, chicory, garlic, spelt, oily fish, pomegranate, kale, kidney beans, lemons, linseed (-oil), mushrooms, nuts, olives (-oil), onions, papaya, spirulina, sweet potatoes, zucchini and most importantly, pure water. You can find tasty and healthy recipes that are easy to prepare from page 79 onward.

It would be easy to get or stay healthy. But the number of doctors who recommend vital mushrooms, cranberries or micro-algae instead of chemical medication is manageable. Since the pharmaceutical industry lures doctors with fat bonuses and trips to the Caribbean intending to burden their patients with expensive chemical bombs.

Aloe vera: beauty & drug candidate against COVID-19

The beneficial succulent is one of more than 400 species in the Aloe genus of the Xanthorrhoeaceae family. It is one of the most researched and used medicinal plants worldwide. Their pharmacological properties and phytochemistry are good documented. (Mukherjee et al. 2014)

Even the beauties of ancient Egypt, Cleopatra and Nefertiti, used the stimulating aloe vera gel of the desert lily for skincare. (Simons 2015)

The main active ingredient in aloe vera is the polysaccharide acemannan in the gel of its thick green leaves. This gel is full of amino acids, sugars, enzymes, hormones, vitamins, minerals and phytochemicals. It's supposedly an effective treatment for skin diseases, mouth problems, microbial growth and digestive disorders.

The human body produces acemannan itself, but only until puberty. It builds this antiviral and antibacterial long-chain type of sugar into all cell membranes. The aloe vera thus sustainably supports the immune system. Acemannan, found in Siberian taiga root and ginseng, also effectively affects the mobility of our joints by providing them with enough synovial fluid.

Aloe vera has already proven against the influenza virus, cytomegalovirus, herpes simplex virus types 1 and 2, poliovirus, varicella-zoster virus, human papillomavirus, feline leukemia virus, the immunodeficiency virus (HIV), including the coronavirus SARS-CoV-1. (Bongo et al., 2020)

When you buy aloe vera juice, better look for organic quality, as it is then generally made from non-irradiated plants and not genetically modified or enriched with fertilizer. Organic aloe vera juice manufacturers do without sweeteners, stabilizers, colorings, preservatives and flavor enhancers.

https://www.globosurfer.com/best-aloe-vera-juices/

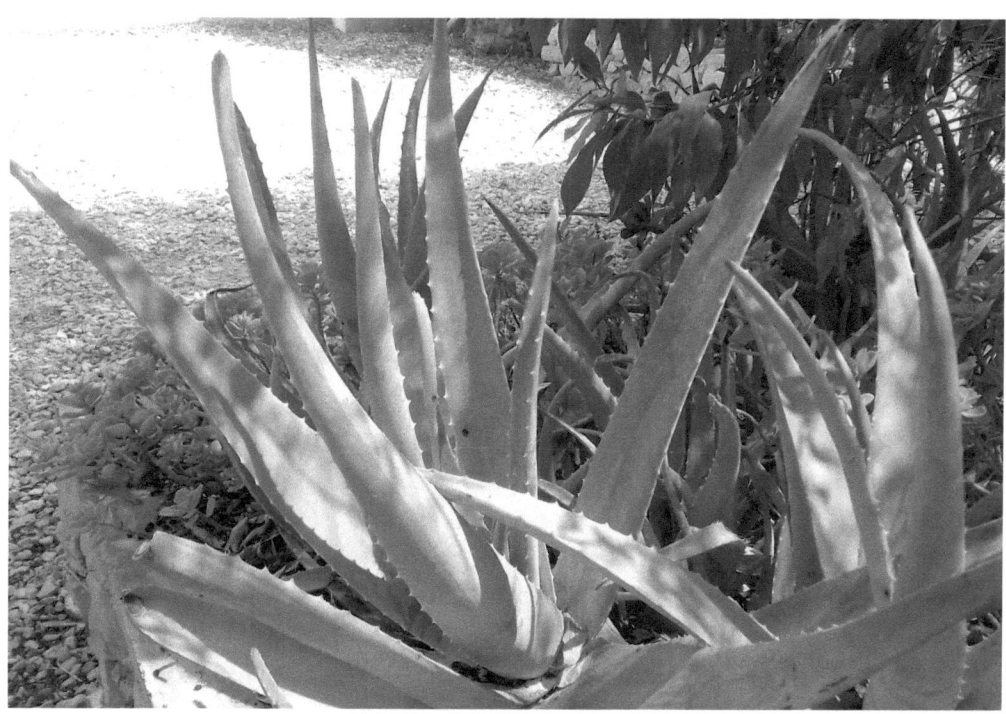

Ashwagandha: the plant that brings you sleep and vitality

The title of the chapter sounds like a contradiction. Withania somnifera (ashwagandha) is called sleep berry or winter cherry in Germany. The word somnifera comes from Latin and means something like bringing sleep. The name ashwagandha comes from Sanskrit. It means the smell of the horse, as the roots smell strongly of a horse. Ashwagandha berries are not used, but roots and leaves. Above all, they reduce stress, increase well-being, promote youthful vitality, improve muscle strength and endurance, and improve general health.

Ashwagandha is used for various disease processes, mainly as a nerve tonic and to nourish the thyroid. Given these facts, countless scientific studies and anti-stress activities proved its potential. Narandra Singh and his Indian colleagues found that Withania somnifera in animal models increased endurance during swimming endurance tests and prevented changes in vitamin C and cortisol levels in the adrenal gland caused by swimming stress.

Pretreatment with ashwagandha showed significant protection against stress-induced gastric ulcers. It has an anti-tumor effect on ovarian cancer and lung adenomas caused by the chemical urethane. In some uterine fibroids and skin cancer cases, long-term treatment with ashwagandha got the condition under control.

Withania somnifera also helps children with poor memory and the elderly with memory loss. It has also been found suitable in neurodegenerative diseases such as Parkinson's, Huntington's, and Alzheimer's.

Ashwagandha is an anti-inflammatory, anti-arthritic agent and has been found useful in clinical cases of rheumatism and osteoarthritis. Large-scale studies are required to prove its clinical efficacy in stress-related and neural disorders and cancer. (Singh et al., 2011)

The Australian researcher Adrian L. Lopresti and his colleagues examined the stress-relieving and pharmacological effects of an ashwagandha extract in stressed healthy adults. The study was a 60-day, randomized, double-blind, placebo-controlled study (Lopresti et al., 2019). In another 16-week, randomized, double-blind, placebo-controlled crossover study, Lopresti and his colleagues examined ashwaganda's effects on fatigue, vitality, and steroid hormones in 57 overweight men aged 40–70 years with mild fatigue. They received an ashwagandha extract (shoden beads with 21 mg of withanolide glycosides per day) or a placebo for eight weeks. Over time, the subjects reported improvements in fatigue, vitality, and sexual and psychological well-being. Ashwagandha intake was associated with an 18% greater increase in DHEA-S and a 14.7% greater increase in testosterone compared to placebo. They also developed more muscle mass and had increased strength values. In addition, they recorded an increase in loss of body fat. (Lopresti et al., 2019)

It would be interesting to investigate more broadly and regardless of gender. In the meantime, we better test ourselves whether the sleeping berries can help us fall asleep and bring new momentum again. Children could also benefit from the herb, as it relieves anxiety and stress and can make Ritalin dispensable. But even adults shouldn't exceed 5 g (1 teaspoon) daily. And those who suffer from autoimmune diseases such as lupus, rheumatism or MS should be careful. Because, like tomatoes and eggplants, ashwagandha belongs to the nightshade family. And in autoimmune diseases, it could increase levels of inflammation in the body.

Personal experience: After consuming a teaspoon of ashwagandha powder in my cereal daily for a few months, I stopped using it. But after a few weeks, I started to feel drained, so I put it back on and had more energy and was able to sleep better.

Astragalus membranaceus activates the immune system

Traditional Chinese medicine (TCM) uses the rejuvenating and life-prolonging root mostly with other energizing and blood-forming natural substances, such as the goji berry (see page 38 f.). Many health benefits ascribe to the astragalus root: it strengthens the immune system, prevents premature aging, has an anti-inflammatory effect and helps with fatigue, allergies and colds. TCM also uses the root against heart problems, diabetes, and liver diseases, even chronic hepatitis. It protects the liver and kidneys, slows down protein loss through the urine (proteinuria) and moderates fibrotic kidney destruction by inhibiting the proliferation of connective tissue fibers. The astragalus root helps reduce damage from kidney infections. And it reduces blood lipids and blood pressure. All in all, it supports the elimination organs as a versatile tonic.

During tick season, astragalus taken daily can repel ticks. Because:

The root changes the body odor, making it uncomfortable for ticks.

Echinacea: the barrier against infection

The purple coneflower is one of the most carefully studied potent medicinal plants. A considerable body of research demonstrates echinacea's immune-stimulating properties. As early as 1885, Dr H.C.F. Meyer was committed to echinacea as a blood purifier. But not until the 1950s and 1960s did German scientists begin to research the medicinal properties of the plant. Since then, the active ingredient in the purple coneflower treats colds. Numerous naturopathic doctors recommend echinacea preparations to support the immune system.

Johanna Signer and her colleagues from Spiez Laboratory in Switzerland found that E. purpurea and E. angustifolia can prevent Sars-CoV-2 infection in humans. The product Echinaforce® exhibits virucidal activity against four coronaviruses in vitro upon direct contact in suspension. (Signer 2020)

Canadian Monique Aucoin and her numerous international research colleagues found that echinacea supplementation can help with symptoms of acute respiratory infections (ARI) and the common cold, particularly when given at the first sign of infection. (Aucoin et al., 2020)

Echinacea we can also take during the winter months as it reduces cold symptoms by more than half and shortens the duration by a day and a half.

Goji berries make you mentally fit, calm, happy and content

Sweet and sour fruits grow on the 2-3 meter high shrub, which is called wolfberry (Lycium barbarum) in German-speaking countries and are incorrectly described as poisonous. The Tibetans call them "lucky berries". They are traded worldwide as a superfood and cultivated extensively in Central Asia. However, you can also easily grow healthy fruits in your garden.

The US researchers Harunobu Amagase and Dwight M. Nance could demonstrate the positive effects of a standardized goji juice (Lycium barbarum) in a randomized, double-blind, placebo-controlled clinical study with 34 participants. They found notable differences between day 1 and day 15 in the Goji group in terms of increased scores for energy levels, athletic performance, sleep quality, ease of awakening, ability to focus on activities, mental acuity, calm and feelings of good health, happiness and luck. Goji juice also significantly reduced fatigue and stress and improved the regularity of gastrointestinal function. (2008)

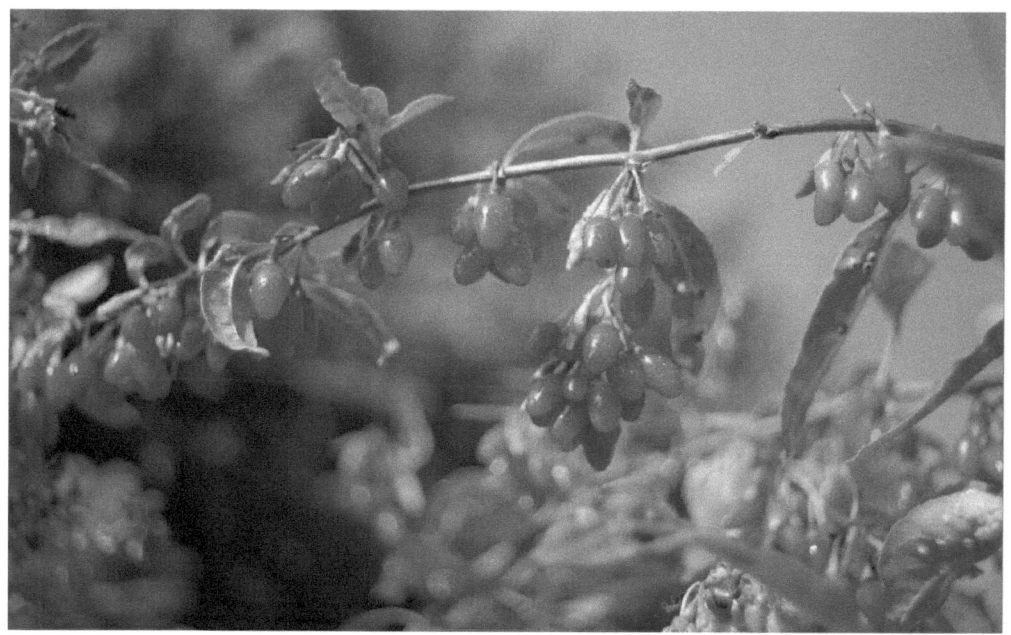

In a 4-week animal study at Washington State University, Yifei Kang and her colleagues could demonstrate improved gastrointestinal functions after chemically induced ulcerative colitis (chronic inflammation of the large intestine) by administering 1% Lycium barbarum to the diet. Also, the goji berry supplementation avoided a 30% mortality rate caused by DSS-induced colitis. (Kang et al., 2017)

Grapefruit seed extract (GKE) kills or deactivates SARS-CoV-2

A grapefruit seed extract has long been considered an insider tip against bacteria, fungi and viruses. As early as 1980, the physician and immunobiologist Dr Jacob Harich observed that the grapefruit seeds on his compost heap hardly rotted. They appeared to be resistant to mold, putrefactive bacteria, viruses, and parasites. Through this goodness of fate, Harich discovered the natural healing power of grapefruit seed extract. The bioflavonoids in the core of the grapefruit protect against harmful influences. Harich and other researchers concluded that these secondary plant substances inherent in the fruit stone, could also provide a protective mechanism in humans. After all, some of my readers report that drinking a few drops of grapefruit seed extract diluted in a glass of water stops diarrhea or flu and cures eczema or skin fungal infections.

The effect of GKE on Avian Influenza Virus (AIV), Newcastle Disease Virus (NDV), Infectious Bursal Disease Virus (IBDV), Salmonella Infantis (SI) and Escherichia coli (EC) is document already in international studies.

Researchers at Utah State University and Northwestern University, led by Mark Cannon, found visible evidence using electron microscopy that xylitol and grapefruit seed extract counteract the virus. GKE kills the virus while xylitol prevents it from attaching itself to cell walls. The researchers were able to show that SARS-CoV-2 viruses are outside the cell and in no way ashered, thus preventing infection.

Researchers tested the response of SARS-CoV-2 virus titers and LRV (Leishmania RNA virus) to a single concentration of Xlear nasal spray. After a contact time of 25 minutes, the nasal spray significantly reduced the virus. This study is the latest in a series of studies concluding that Xlear is effective against SARS-CoV-2.

Personal experience: I used to use a few drops of GKE in a glass of water after accidentally eating spoiled or poisonous food. After a single episode of diarrhea, stomach pains went away. Today I use CS (colloidal silver).

Ginger: The hot rhizome inhibits the multiplication of viruses

Ginger (Zingiber officinale) is a distinctive spice and medicinal plant that has been used for thousands of years to relieve pain and inflammation. We use ginger for many conditions, including colds, nausea, arthritis, migraines, and high blood pressure. Arab traders controlled the ginger market for centuries in the Middle Ages. Therefore, a pound of ginger had cost as much as a sheep and were considered a real luxury good (Bode and Dong, 2011). Yasmin Anum Mohd Yusof regards the use of 6-gingerol, found notably in fresh ginger, to be a safe means of preventing and treating chronic diseases (2015). It is arguably due to its antioxidant activity.

Ginger's anti-COVID-19 effects benefited the Nigerian state of Enugu residents during the pandemic. Ginger alone or combined with other vitamin C fortified plants such as bitter kola, garlic, turmeric, and lime could be a therapy for COVID-

40

19 or prophylaxis in Enugu-Nigeria, and around the world to eliminate the coronavirus. (Obeta, 2020)

Jung San Chang and his Taiwanese research colleagues tested the effect of hot water extracts from fresh and dried ginger on HRSV (human respiratory syncytial virus). Only fresh ginger is effective against HRSV-induced plaque formation on airway epithelium by blocking viral attachment and internalization. Fresh ginger was more effective when given before viral inoculation. (Chang et al., 2013)

In addition to the antimicrobial effect, ginger promotes fat digestion and increases the formation of gastric juice, saliva, and bile. It also stimulates blood circulation and turns the cycle on. Its pungent substances warm you, especially in the winter, in a soothing tea that prevents colds. In the summer, a couple of fresh ginger slices in water make a refreshing drink.

Traditional Chinese Medicine (TCM) and Indian Ayurveda have been using ginger root for hair loss for thousands of years. It stimulates blood flow in the scalp. This improved blood supply can activate the hair follicles and restore hair growth.

The fiery root contains a lot of potassium and vitamin C, phosphorus, and riboflavin. The secondary plant substances gingerol and zingiberol, specific to ginger, are particularly effective. Together with other active ingredients, these substances ensure that ginger can stop hair loss and stimulate new hair growth.

Hair oil against hair loss

2 thumb-sized pieces of peeled and freshly grated ginger
3 tablespoons sesame, linseed or olive oil
1 teaspoon lemon juice
1 teaspoon instant coffee

Mix all the ingredients and massage the mixture into your scalp using circular motions. Cover with a plastic bag and a towel. Rinse well after 15 to 30 minutes.

41

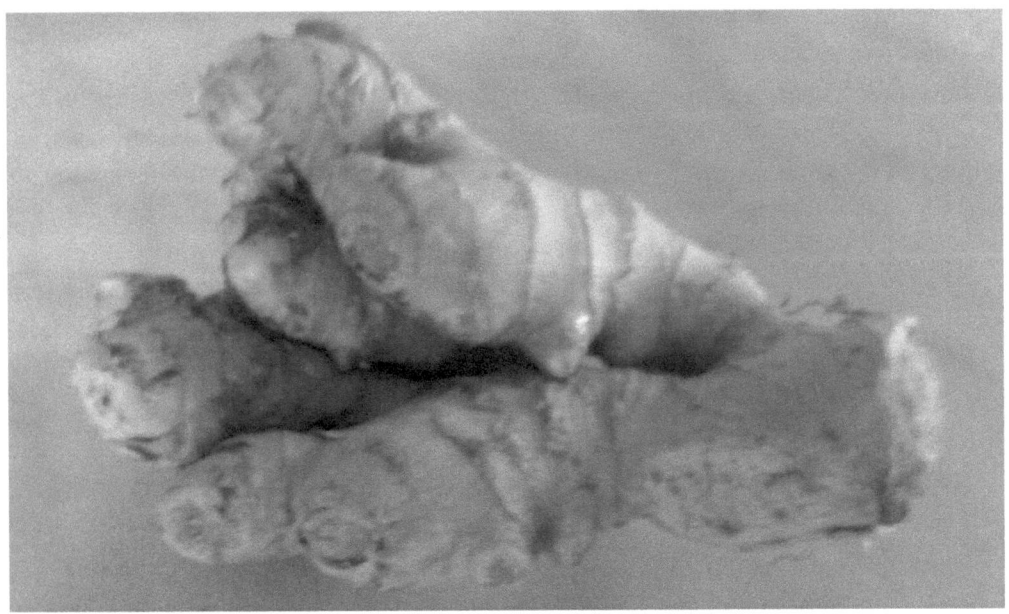

Garlic fights coronavirus infections

Garlic (Allium sativum), the leek plant found around the globe today, is used as a flavoring and antimicrobial and anti-diarrheal agent. Its characteristic scent comes from the substances alliin and allicin. These prevent reactions in the body that lead to inflammation. Garlic compounds even reduce life-threatening inflammation like dengue virus infection and oxidative stress. (Hall et al., 2017)

Garlic extracts also have an inhibitory effect on the infectious bronchitis virus (IBV) in the chick embryo. The researchers evaluated the groups treated with garlic extract eight hours after the virus challenge to show at which stage of the virus infection the garlic extract was effective. The result showed a possible effect on the virus in the replication phase. (Mohajer Shojai et al., 2016)

Incidentally, the infectious bronchitis virus is a coronavirus! The available vaccines against IBV are said to be unable to cover new variants. So why not recommend garlic to people to fight a coronavirus infection associated with increased inflammation. In addition, the active phytochemicals in garlic can lower cholesterol and prevent blood clots and the hardening of the arteries. It relaxes blood vessels, reducing their bursting with just 1-2 garlic cloves per day. It is best to grate them or press them through the press and let them sit for 5 to 10 minutes before eating. Thereby the active components combine, by which sulphur compounds can develop. (Kreutzer and Larsen, 2018)

However, eating fresh garlic on an empty stomach can cause discomfort. But garlic isn't just good for your health. It is also said to improve your appearance significantly and to work against belly fat. Black garlic (BG), obtained through fermentation, is particularly beneficial. We receive it from fresh garlic (Allium sativum L.) that has been fermented at a controlled high temperature (60-90 °C) and controlled high humidity (80-90%) for a specific period. As compared to fresh garlic, BG does not develop a strongly offensive aroma due to the reduced allicin content. It is also better tolerated. Allicin was converted into significantly higher antioxidant compounds in the BG by fermentation. These include bioactive alkaloids and flavonoids. Black garlic is anti-inflammatory, anti-cancer and anti-allergic. For type 2 diabetes, BG may be more effective than regular garlic.

Jingbo Liu and his US research colleagues studied the clinical effects of black garlic in 120 patients with congestive heart failure caused by coronary artery disease. Garlic treatment improved heart function compared to the placebo group. Circulating antioxidant levels were also higher in the BG group than in the placebo group. (Liu et al., 2018)

Turmeric may make its mark as a COVID-19 prophylactic

Curcumin, a bioactive compound in turmeric, exerts multiple pharmacological effects and is often used in foods and traditional medicines. It is, therefore, suitable for the prevention of COVID-19, according to Rajesh K. Thimmulappa and his Indian research colleagues. Because curcumin exerts antiviral activity against many enveloped viruses, including SARS-CoV-2. It does it through these mechanisms: direct interaction with viral membrane proteins, disruption of the viral envelope, inhibition of viral proteases and triggering of host antiviral responses. Curcumin also protects against fatal pneumonia and acute lung failure. It is safe and well-tolerated in both healthy and sick people. (Thimmulappa et al., 2021)

The authors, therefore, believe that this accumulated evidence could position curcumin as a potential prophylactic therapeutic for COVID-19 in the clinic and public health setting. So it is wise to spice your food with turmeric.

Neroli oil activates the pineal gland, which slows the aging process

Neroli oil derives from the blossom of the bitter orange or Citrus aurantium. The floral, fresh and lovely sweet-scented oil has a relaxing, anticonvulsant and stimulating effect. It is perfect for aromatherapy. Since neroli oil also stimulates the pineal gland, it promotes our physical and mental health and increases our intuition, the so-called gut feeling.

The epiphysis called the pineal gland because it resembles the shape of the pine cones. It regulates our internal clock and sleep and, as already mentioned, increases our inner senses. When the pineal gland weakens, the physical and psychological aging process begins. That is associated with problems falling asleep and staying asleep. The epiphysis converts the serotonin produced in the intestine and the nerve cells of the brain during the day into melatonin in the dark of the night. Serotonin is one of the happiness hormones because it has a relaxing and mood-enhancing effect. The second hormone promotes falling asleep, regulates sleeping patterns, regenerates cell damage during the night and protects our cells as a powerful antioxidant. According to studies, melatonin has an even more powerful antioxidant effect than the synthetic antioxidant DMSO, often used for therapeutic purposes.

Due to our modern way of life, the pineal gland has atrophied in the course of evolution from approximately 3 centimeters to a few millimeters. Fluoride is particularly destructive but also hormones, mercury, tobacco, alcohol, caffeine, and sugar can cause calcification of the pineal gland. Therefore, regular detoxification measures are crucial: with quality spring water, chlorella, spirulina, psyllium husk powder, bentonite, zeolite and other clay minerals. It is also important to relieve the liver with bitter substances such as dandelion or plantain. And just as you activate the thymus function of making T-cells by tapping as the monkeys do, you can stimulate the pineal gland function. Namely, when you sing. The vibration of singing stimulates your epiphysis. But in particular, you energize the pineal gland and thus your intuition with the essential neroli oil. It is best to inhale it during meditation in the sun. So you have the triple effect: fragrance, relaxation and solar energy.

Neroli oil has a calming effect on the nervous system. It also reduces fears. And that is vital for survival, especially in troubled times.

www.zentrum-der-gesundheit.de/bibliothek/koerper/koerperfunktionen/zirbeldruese
https://www.decleor.com/en/oil-effects/moisture-lock/neroli.html

Oregano Oil: A powerful natural antibiotic

Due to its very high carvacrol content, oregano oil is one of the most potent essential oils. Because of its antibacterial, antiviral, fungicidal and anti-parasitic properties, oregano oil has a strong disinfecting effect. And unlike chemical antibiotics, no resistance develops. It helps against inflammation of the airways and lymphatic system and loosens mucus in respiratory diseases, such as bronchitis and whooping cough. In addition, it promotes blood circulation and relieves pain. But oregano oil is not only effective against colds, candida, bacterial overgrowth of the small intestine (SIBO=small intestinal bacterial overgrowth), fungal diseases, acne and gingivitis. It can also treat or prevent diabetes, cancer and other diseases.

Katerina Spyridopoulou and her colleagues analyzed the chemical composition of the essential oil Origanum onites (OOEO = Origanum onites essential oil). Oregano primarily grows in Greece, Turkey and Sicily. For the first time, the researchers demonstrated the anti-cancer potential of orally administered OOEO in the test tube and the living organism. The oregano oil stopped the growth of colon tumors. This documentary is especially gratifying for cancer patients since the plant extract helps people suffering from RNA viruses but in much larger numbers from cancer.

Please be extremely careful with the dosage because the oil is very spicy. So use no more than 2 to 3 drops in some water or tea.

Polyporus: Antibiotic & stimulant for the heart, kidneys, skin and hair

This medicinal mushroom is not only blessed with many pores but also with a lot of healing potential. In China, it is considered the oldest natural antibiotic. That also seems to be confirmed by the mummy from the Ötztal Glacier. Five thousand years ago, Ötzi had two related mushrooms from the Porlinge family in his shaman pouch.

Polyporus is one of the few natural remedies to stimulate lymph flow. It, therefore, supports our lymphatic system – the body's waste disposal system – in draining water. That relieves the immune system and lowers kidney-related high blood pressure (2nd value), which should not be higher than 80. Polyporus counteracts unsightly swellings on the hands and ankles. It beautifies the complexion and stimulates hair growth.

The medicinal mushroom is effective against the multi-resistant pus pathogen Staphylococcus aureus (MRSA hospital germ). Ulrike Lindequist and her German research colleagues were able to demonstrate this. They summarized the beneficial activities of various fungi on gut microbiota (formerly called gut flora) via inhibition of externally acting pathogens and thereby improving host health (Lindequist et al. 2005). See also Grunewald et al., 2018.

Polyporus also helps with bladder or kidney inflammation and kidney stones with painful urination and blood in the urine due to its flushing effect. Furthermore, the versatile medicinal mushroom protects the liver, strengthens the stomach, loosens muscle tissue, strengthens the respiratory tract, and expands the bronchi in chronic bronchitis and asthma. For lung problems, the polyporus is used together with the reishi and the cordyceps medicinal mushroom.

The polyporus umbellatus inhibits tumor cell proliferation and promotes the programmed cell death of tumor cells. Xiao-Lang Tan and her Chinese research colleagues proved this in test tube studies and living organisms. They concluded that polyporus umbellatus might play a potential role in human breast cancer control and represent a therapeutic strategy for breast cancer suppression. (Tan et al., 2016)

The fungus for skin and blood vessels also helps with:
– Cancer (lung, liver, prostate, leukemia, sarcoma)
– Liver diseases
– Water excretion without increased potassium excretion
– Lowering blood fat and strengthening the heart
– Immune stimulation in infections
– Blood pressure regulation
https://www.mycomedica.eu/polyporus.html#cookie-lista

Quickly clear of COVID-19 and no severe symptoms with quercetin

Based on the antiviral, anticoagulant, anti-inflammatory and antioxidant properties of quercetin, Francesco Di Pierro and his international research colleagues hypothesized the following: 21 patients with mild COVID-19 treated with quercetin Phytosome® (QP), a novel bioavailable form of quercetin, may have a shorter time to virus clearance, milder symptoms, and a higher likelihood of benign earlier disease resolution. The results also showed that after one week of treatment, 16 patients in the QP group tested negative for SARS-CoV-2, and 12 patients had all symptoms alleviated. Of the 21 patients who did not receive a QP, two patients tested SARS-CoV-2 negative and four patients partially improved their symptoms.

Therefore, I consider the consumption of the flavonoid quercetin, which naturally occurs primarily in capers, red onions and grapes or red wine and green tea. And not only in the case of a positive corona test. If I tested positive, I'd take one 500 mg quercetin capsule three times a day for six weeks and incorporate the above foods into my diet. The following link shows what you should know about the uses and contraindications.

https://orthopaedie-innsbruck.at/quercetin-6685#Interactions
https://www.medicalnewstoday.com/articles/324170

Shiitake Mushroom: nerve and gut-soothing source of vitamin D

Due to its impressive healing effects, the king of medicinal mushrooms has the highest efficiency of all medicinal mushrooms. In China and Japan, the shiitake mushroom (*Lentinula edodes* or *Lentinus edodes*) has been a solid part of the medicine cabinet for thousands of years. It provides firm connective tissue and acts as an immune stabilizer. It also inhibits tumors. Traditional Chinese Medicine uses the spicy-tasting medicinal mushroom primarily for arteriosclerosis, diabetes, measles, hepatitis and anti-aging. You can also use it for high blood pressure, joint inflammation or rheumatic complaints.

In Japan, the shiitake mushroom is known for its antitumor effects and has even been approved as a drug against stomach cancer. The ingredient lentinan helps the body locate and destroy cancer cells faster. Pressed juice from the shiitake shall inhibit the uncontrolled growth of tumor cell lines. The Japanese also recommend it for gout, stomach ulcers, neuralgia and constipation.

Emma J. Murphy and her Irish research colleagues could demonstrate the immune system-modifying and lung cell-protecting effects of different shiitake extracts, which may also be of positive importance for possible COVID-19 therapeutics against cytokine storm. (Murphy et al., 2020)

Many people in Central and Northern Europe suffer from a vitamin D deficiency, which is often the cause of chronic illness. Luckily, the shiitake mushroom is an excellent source of vitamin D. Deficient people can benefit from the regular intake of mushrooms cultivated in the open air. Further from fatty fish and the less enjoyable cod liver oil. Finnish researchers determined in a study that many mushrooms, including shiitake, have an enormous ergosterol content. Thus, they can be essential sources of vitamin D. Since ergosterol is the precursor (provitamin) of vitamin D2 (ergocalciferol) it can be photochemically converted by UV radiation (e. g. sunlight). https://de.wikipedia.org/wiki/Ergosterol

Officially, the daily requirement of vitamin D is given as 600 to 800 IU, unofficially as 4,000 to 8,000 IU. Studies have now shown that 100 grams of shiitake mushrooms, which initially contained only 100 IU (2.5 μg) of vitamin D, contain a full 46,000 IE after the researchers dried them in the sun for six hours each day for two days. That means:

2 to 10 grams of shiitake mushrooms exposed to the sun would be enough to meet the daily vitamin D requirement.

Since you do not know how mushrooms were grown when you buy them, you can dry them in the sun afterwards to turn them into a better source of vitamin D. And with it, you can then strengthen your immune system and prevent allergies, candida, flu, colds, cancer and other immune deficiency diseases. So there is some evidence that the healing effect of shiitake is based principally on stimulating the immune system. Bacteria, viruses, fungi and parasites can be held down by the body's defense mechanisms, mainly through its polysaccharides. That includes the beta-glucan lentinan, which according to American and Asian scientists, is one of the most effective activators of the immune system.

zentrum-der-gesundheit.de/ernaehrung/Lebensmittel/pilze-uebersicht/shiitake-pilze

https://www.healthline.com/nutrition/shiitake-mushrooms

M. Gordon and her US research colleagues conducted two placebo-controlled studies with a total of 98 patients at the San Francisco General Hospital. The participants had an HIV positive test, a CD4 level of 200 to 500 cells. They were between 18 and 60 years of age and without current opportunistic infections. In the first study, ten patients received 2, 5 or 10 mg lentinan or a placebo intravenously once a week for eight weeks. The second study had two groups: 20 patients received 1 or 5 mg lentinan intravenously twice a week for 12 weeks. Ten patients received a placebo. The patients in the study had a trend towards increasing levels of T helper cells (CD4 lymphocytes). Some had neutrophil activity. (Gordon et al. 1998)

Neutrophils are the most common white blood cells, known as the body police force. This study also confirmed the superior lentinan tolerability in European subjects, as observed in Japanese cancer patients. It would certainly be worth doing a large long-term study of shiitake mushrooms. As long as there is no scientific interest in this, I advise you to become active yourself and to use the tasty mushroom more often in your kitchen because our own experiences are what create knowledge. You can find my delicious creations in the recipe section.

Incidentally, you can purchase the organic shiitake culture for the cellar, greenhouse or garden by mail order and grow the medicinal mushroom yourself. Since the mushroom growth in shiitake activates by vibration, the culture usually comes to you with mushrooms.

As I already mentioned, if you let them dry in the sun for two days before eating, the already considerable vitamin D content increases. Therefore, you better activate the shiitake culture that came with the cover sheet and Mycil-inoculated substrate as soon as you receive it. All you then need is a coaster or flat stone with an average of 40 cm. It can be grown indoors or in a greenhouse all year round. Since the culture needs light and temperatures between +14°C and +22°C for fungal growth, you can do it on the balcony, terrace or in the garden at higher temperatures. Outdoors, place the culture in a shady, damp place as sheltered as possible from the wind, preferably under a deciduous tree or bush.

Internal Cleansing Mushroom helps with:

– the lowering of cholesterol levels
– poor immune system and infections as well as prevention
– high blood pressure, arteriosclerosis and heart attack prophylaxis
– tumor diseases of the digestive organs, the lungs and the blood
– diabetes, allergies, circulatory disorders and much more more
– detox cure, since it has an antibacterial and antioxidant effect
– cancer therapies

Thapsia garganica: The carrot of death kills cancer and COVID-19

A further natural agent that inhibits SARS-CoV-2, influenza A virus, and other respiratory viruses is the phytochemical thapsigargin. It is extracted from the yellow flowering *Thapsia garganica* plant. You can use it prophylactically to prevent an infection or as a therapeutic agent for the disease.

We find thapsigargin in the roots and fruits of the *Thapsia L* species. Farmers from the western Mediterranean and central and southern Portugal fear for their livestock because of the plant poison that flowers here from April to June/July (I shot the pic on April 30). However, folk medicine treats rheumatic diseases, lung ailments and female infertility. Here, the statement of Paracelsus applies: "All things are poison, and nothing is without poison; the dose alone makes the poison.

About thirty years ago, Agata Jaskulska and her Polish research colleagues found the following: Due to the biological activity and molecular mechanisms of thapsigargin action and in the context of the development process in the synthesis of less toxic thapsigargin derivatives, the death carrot is suitable as a novel anticancer drug. (Jaskulska et al., 1990)

Therefore, the tumor-promoting sesquiterpene lactone thapsigargin protecting against predators, can save people from death. The dose makes the poison.

Sarah Al-Betai and her predominantly British research colleagues showed in a series of COVID-19 patients with low to medium risk: An intranasal combination therapy led to rapid clinical improvement with repeated intranasal swab tests using PCR. According to the authors, this discovery could have significant implications for the treatment of future epidemics and pandemics. Thapsigargin can be used to prevent infection and as a therapeutic agent in the disease. For example, if used once, it can prevent the virus from spreading further for up to 48 hours.

Since the antiviral agent is stable in an acidic environment such as the stomach, you can take it orally. There is no need for injections or hospital stays. The researchers also report that it is insensitive to virus resistance. And:

Thapsigargin is "at least a hundred times more effective than current antiviral options".

https://www.nottingham.ac.uk/news/thapsigargin-COVID-19

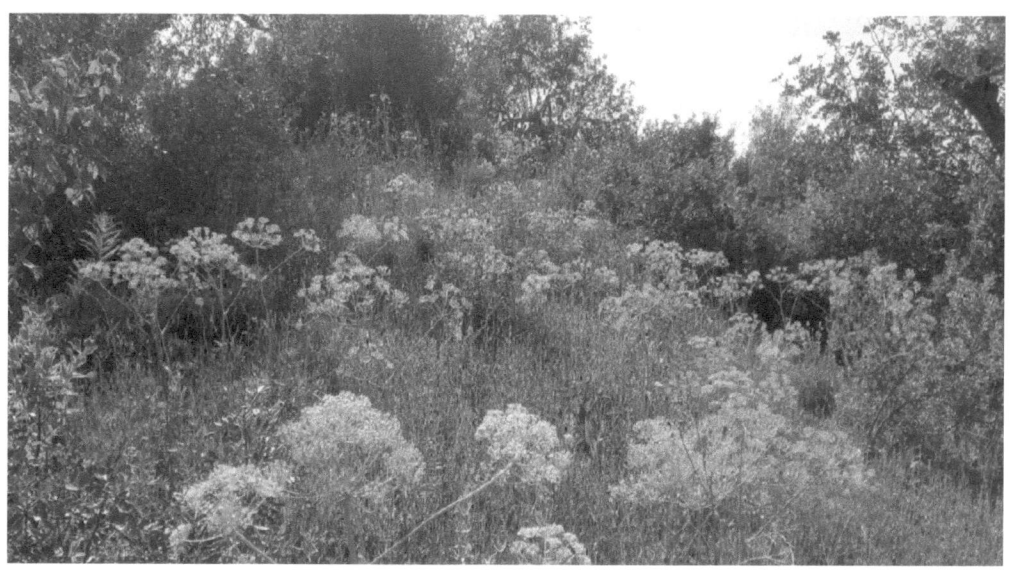

Working groups from the pharmacological and virological institutes at JLU Giessen published their work on September 22nd, 2021. They found that the antiviral effect of thapsigargin already occurs at low concentrations. "Thapsigargin reduces viral titers by a factor of 100 to 1000. A single dose is enough to stop virus replication for up to three days completely." And:

Thapsigargin is ten times more effective than remdesivir in SARS-CoV-2

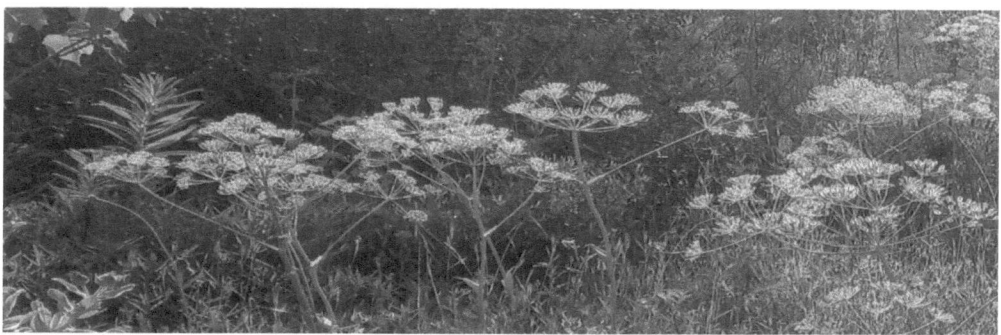

https://www.giessener-anzeiger.de/lokales/stadt-giessen/nachrichten-giessen/thapsigargin-hemmt-vermehrung-von-coronaviren_24519717

IV. MODERN DISEASE: BODY ACIDITY

If you are acidic, you have too many acids or too few bases in your body. Medically, it is called acidosis and can be detected in urine or blood and is less expensive to diagnose with a scalar wave analysis. The latter bio-resonance procedure, to record the parameters of bodily fluids, bones, tissue, etc., is described in the chapter *Scalar wave analysis - a breakthrough in medical practice.*

How does acidosis develop and manifest itself?

If the pH value in the blood falls below 7.35, we speak of acidosis. A diet high in animal foods is often the cause. However, certain medications and diseases can also trigger hyperacidity.

The biochemical process of eating requires us to absorb the nutritional elements from food to keep us alive. To use these elements, they must burn in our bodies. However, this chemical reaction, or oxidation, produces by-products such as carbon dioxide and hydrogen ions, also a variety of acids that the body can no longer process. He excretes these products, which a few are harmful, via the liver, intestines, skin and kidneys. The hydrogen ions combine with the oxygen and eliminate with the urine.

If these hydrogen ions - the dirt in the blood - remain in large quantities, acidosis develops. The more hydrogen ions remain in the blood more oxygen is needed to bind them. It deprives the body of oxygen. Signs of this are blue lips. If the blood plasma is overly acidic, the body tires with the slightest exertion and energy slacks. Even apathy can set in. Headaches or susceptibility to inflammation also occur. If this condition worsens, diseases such as diabetes or osteoporosis develop. That is why one speaks of hyperacidity as a breeding ground for disease.

Malnutrition, stress and lack of exercise are the chief causes of acidification of body fluids.

If the supply is not sufficient of sodium, potassium and magnesium in the food, a tendency to acidosis develops. To maintain the acid-base balance, it is thus crucial to consume large amounts of these minerals. However, since the Western diet consists chiefly of chemically treated and processed foods, one cannot hope to obtain these alkalizing minerals from the ordinary diet. You can counteract hyperacidity with targeted nutrition and dietary supplements such as spirulina, cereal grasses or wild herbs from meadows away from traffic and by eliminating stress.

Acid-forming diet and lifestyle

It would be easy to get your acid-base balance under control or keep it in balance. If you were to make 80% of your daily diet alkaline and only 20% acidic, you would not even have to do without acidifiers such as meat, grains or sweets completely. But the modern diet and lifestyle can very easily lead to over-acidification of the organism. Today we sit for hours in front of the TV and PC or use the cell phone. It exposes us to a lot of electrosmog. Stress acids add, especially if we don't balance with meditation, yoga, contemplation, etc. The latter procedures are crucial if you feel anxious, grumpy, worried or plagued by negative thoughts.

But also, if you overdo it with sports activities or physical work, you form acids in the body; also with alcoholic beverages, coffee, nicotine, medicines and dental poisons (mercury, palladium).

Regarding nutrition, animal proteins such as meat, sausage, fish, milk and soy products lead to acidosis. The latter contain hardly any healthy nutrients. But also legumes, except for white beans, lead to acid formation. We also better eat bread, pasta and pastries in moderation. Ready meals and light and diet products also over-acidify and harm us as they confuse the body with artificial substances in the long run. Snacks like protein bars or microwave popcorn do more harm than they promise. The former can cause edema, abdominal pain and constipation. And the butter flavor diacetyl in the microwave corn kernels carries the risk of bronchial inflammation to the point of scarring the lung tissue, which can make a lung transplant necessary. So we better buy corn kernels in the health food store and pop them in the pot. However, diacetyl also flavors margarine, frying oils, other snacks and diet products. The ACE drinks, whose name derived from the vitamins A, C and E, are also life-threatening.

Cola, sodas and many other carbonated drinks contain a lot of sugar. Therefore, they are strongly acid-forming and promote obesity. The latter also applies to instant soups, broths and sauces. Almost all of them contain synthetic preservatives, colorings, flavor enhancers such as glutamate (E621), often only declared as aroma, seasoning or yeast extract) and sweeteners such as saccharin, cyclamate or aspartame. The latter suspected neurotoxin is also known as NutraSweet, E951 or Candarel. If you cannot do without sweeteners, you are better off with the stevia rebaudiana plant and boiling down the leaves to make your liquid sweetness. Commercial stevia sweetener, liquid, as a powder or tablet, is known under the additive E960. (Simonsohn, 2010)

The food commonly eaten today is no longer a living substance beneficial to the organism. Digesting and metabolizing highly processed foods produce large amounts of acids, toxins, and metabolic end products that overwhelm the body's self-regulating systems. Therefore, you'd better provide body cleansing every spring and fall described in the following part.

What can baking soda do for our health?

Sodium bicarbonate, also known as sodium hydrogen carbonate or simply baking soda, is a substance that has long been known in the kitchen as baking soda or for cleaning fruits and vegetables. We also use it for many purposes in the household: for drain cleaning, as an odor barrier for carpets or animal hair. Above all, baking soda covers a wide range of applications in medicine.

Family doctors used baking soda to heal sore throats, insect bites, blemished skin, heartburn, nausea, stomach problems, inflammation such as arthritis and other autoimmune diseases.

Generally, it is effective for all diseases based on hyperacidity, as it produces an alkaline environment. By the way, COVID-19 viruses and their mutants don't like it alkaline at all.

Doctors these days are unlikely to recommend this cheap wonder drug to you due to conflicts of interest. They also won't tell you that baking soda instantly converts to CO_2 in the stomach, driving bicarbonates into the blood and increasing oxygen levels in body fluids and tissues.

Also, young women seem to protect better with baking soda than with an HPV vaccine. I agree with Leonard Coldwell, author of The Only Answer to Cancer, for whom every vaccination is an assault, sometimes even murder. Gardasil, the HPV vaccine designed to protect against human papillomavirus infection, is the best evidence of this. Numerous dead and neurologically damaged girls prove it. The vaccine is designed to prevent uterine cancer, which is claimed to be caused by the human papillomavirus and can quickly be cured with a few rinses with baking soda. (2017)

Personal experience: Baking soda helps me fall asleep. I also use it in the bath or as a foot bath to deacidify. I also use baking soda and vinegar for baking my quick rolls (see page 97) every week and clean my raw foods by soaking them in apple cider vinegar and baking soda water for about 10 minutes.

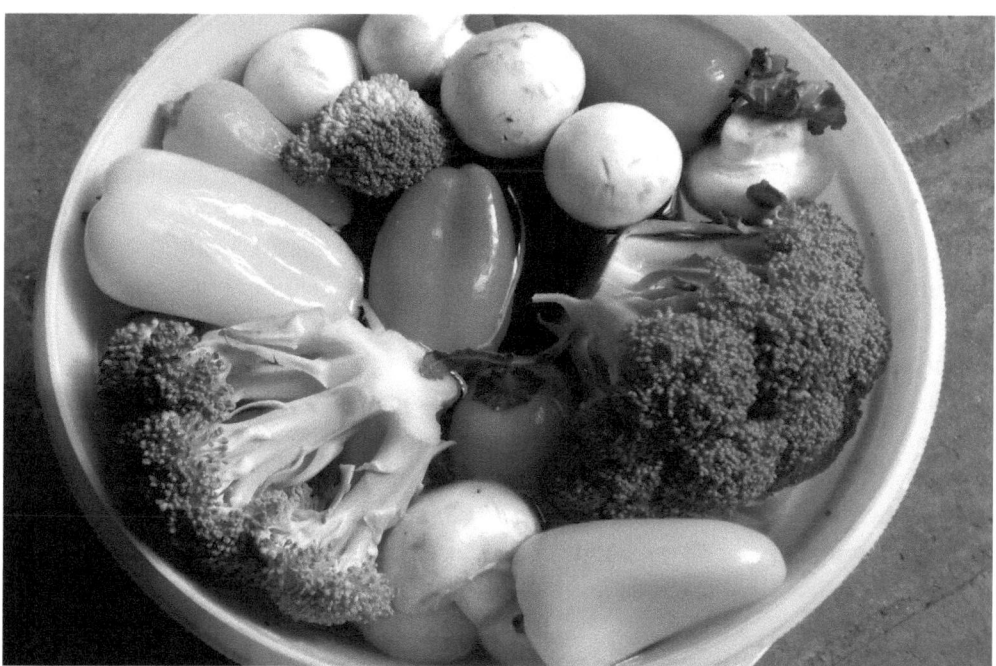

V. SCALAR-WAVE ANALYSIS – BREAKTHROUGH IN MEDICAL DIAGNOSTIC

With scalar waves, we are in a new paradigm in terms of our future regarding different kinds of diagnostics, therapies and medication. This chapter is primarily about identifying hidden diseases or nutrient deficiencies and the associated natural measures for healing or compensating for the deficits.

Can scalar-wave diagnostic revolutionize medicine?

Doctors often have problems diagnosing diseases. If they don't know what to do, they put them into the box 'psychological'. These are often diseases caused by a lack of micro-nutrients or an abundance of micro-organisms. The first we induce when we consume not enough fresh food since heating destroys many vitamins and enzymes. If you do not get the latter bio-catalysts from your food, the pancreas has to generate them, overworking at all times. That's when you also get tired.

The other illness doctors often put into the above box is yeast contagion. If it itches in the warm and humid areas, scalp, eyes, ears, nose, navel or anus, the candida albicans yeast usually takes over. Often after consuming sweets or alcohol. An anti-candida diet and spirulina, hydrogen peroxide (H_2O_2), colloidal silver, or grapefruit seed extract can help. If, after an initial aggravation, the symptoms subside 3-4 days later, you can be almost sure it was candida. But I would refrain from sweets, sweet fruits and white flour products for a few more weeks.

You can also detect an infection by mixing H_2O_2 with water in a spray bottle and spraying it on your body. It foams in the places where the mycosis is. So you can always get your fungal disease under control if you have again consumed too much cake, chocolate or wine. Good luck and perseverance! By the way, I've known about this problem since I was a child. When I scratched my head, my old teacher often called out: Leave the little animals alone!

Modern physics complements the possibilities of allopathic healing

Fortunately, in more than forty years of research, scientists have developed the scalar wave analyzer to determine the health status of patients using bio-resonance.

The bio-resonance procedure assumes that the exchange of information between the body cells can be disturbed or blocked by stressful influences such as chemical substances, environmental toxins, radiation exposure, bacteria and viruses. Health problems can be the result. With the help of magnetic scalar waves, the analysis device can record which stresses apply to the patient. The communication between our cells opens up unimagined healing opportunities.

The studies were thus comprehensive because the common activity values for each component ought to be found according to the biophysical information. The development of bio-resonance devices began in 1980. In 1994 they were recognized as a medical device by the Ministry of Health of the Russian Federation. If you are interested in an apprenticeship, you can get information from the following link of the Institute for Biosensorics and Bioenergetic Environmental Research (IBBU). https://ibbu.at/wp-content/uploads/2021/07/Seminarplan_IBBU_2021_2022_Grundlagen.pdf

Initially, this system was developed to evaluate the health of astronauts on missions and athletes in major competitions. Since then, we have been using it in different areas of health, homeopathy, osteopathy, aesthetics and fitness studios.

The "scalar wave pope" Konstantin Meyl, professor of power electronics at Furtwangen University, is known for his theory of potential vortices and extended field theory. He shows us how modern physics can complement the possibilities of medicine. The central question is where the cell energy comes from and what resonance is. Bio-resonance tests and therapy work with the body's electromagnetic vibrations, i.e. on an energetic level. The knowledge, that living beings emit information or have individual electromagnetic fields is the basis for this diagnosis and therapy.

Studies in biophysics have also shown that metabolic processes in the human body are subject to electromagnetic oscillations. Even organs have an individual energy potential. As in homeopathy, in which the vibrations of certain plants transmit to humans, frequencies in bio-resonance therapy influence processes in the body to change the mind, eliminate toxins and activate the self-healing powers. While working with the bio-resonance scanner, progress studies are convincing and a clear sign of progressive healing and regeneration up to biophysical normality.

The result we get with the test device is roughly comparable to laboratory diagnostics. Instead of taking blood and analyzing it in the laboratory, it carries out a spectral analysis and evaluates the measurement result immediately. With this groundbreaking device, we can detect more than 200 body parameters within 31 selected areas in just under two minutes. It informs about micro-nutrients, acid-base balance, potential allergens, bone density, blood sugar, thyroid values, pollution and much more. The advantage over blood tests is that an error such as contamination of blood samples mixed-up is impossible. And you save a lot of time and money.

Kalzium	1,219 - 3,021	1,358	
Eisen	1,151 - 1,847	0,751	
Zink	1,143 - 1,989	1,212	
Selen	0,847 - 2,045	0,729	
Phosphor	1,195 - 2,134	1,493	
Kalium	0,689 - 0,987	0,864	
Magnesium	0,568 - 0,992	0,551	
Kupfer	0,474 - 0,749	0,206	
Kobalt	2,326 - 5,531	3,238	
Mangan	0,497 - 0,879	0,828	
Jod	1,421 - 5,490	4,733	
Nickel	2,462 - 5,753	5,541	
Fluor	1,954 - 4,543	3,81	
Molybdän	0,938 - 1,712	1,064	
Vanadium	1,019 - 3,721	2,939	
Zinn	1,023 - 7,627	5,88	

In the above analysis via Bioscan by non-medical practitioner Angelika Pape four years ago, my iron content was 0.751; copper was 0.206. Since cooking with a cast-iron pan, the iron level is now within normal limits. Since I put copper coins in the kettle, the copper level has almost as you can see in the results of the scalar wave device used by naturopath Sergio de Jesus. It is called the Analisador Ressonância Magnética Quantica. The trolls of the disease industry slander bio-resonance as nonsense. But how is it then that the values correlate with physical reality? How can it be nonsense if e. g. my bad eyesight is recognized? In the middle is the normal range.

Hierro	1,151 - 1,847	1,372
Cobre	0,474 - 0,749	0,37
Fatiga visual	2,017 - 5,157	8,34

IV. DETOXIFYING EFFECTIVELY: HOW WE GET RID OF ACIDS

The modern plague of body acidification is the cause of most health problems. Our organism deposits acid residues in the blood vessels. They lead to narrowing and, as a result, high blood pressure. They can even trigger a heart attack or stroke.

To strengthen your immune system, it is crucial that you sporadically eliminate harmful substances and acids accumulated in the body. Because, with all the loaded garbage, our cells cannot process nutrients. Spring and fall are the best times for detoxification. But you can also detoxify by regularly consuming certain foods, as you can read in the following chapter.

When you cleanse the body, drink plenty of pure water and exercise in the fresh air. Sauna sessions are also helpful. You can find out, how to Stop der Azidose, Allergien und Haarausfall in the book by Halima Neumann. (2008)

The best foods to detox

If you want to cleanse your body naturally, dare to try a regenerating regimen to flush toxins out of your body. By detoxifying your body, i.e. eliminating the accumulated pollutants, you relieve your detoxification organs: i.e. the liver, kidneys, intestines, lymphatic system and skin.
If you are often tired or suffer from frequent colds, cleansing your body through a selected diet can get you going again.

These include sour apples, artichokes, avocados, berries, fennel, leafy greens, green leafy vegetables, green tea, kale, ginger, carrots, potatoes, c, herbs, papaya, beetroot, salads, asparagus, spinach, sweet potatoes, water, and Savoy.

I prefer to eat sweet fruits such as bananas, dates and figs in moderation because of the sugar. Sour varieties like berries, grapefruit, and lemon are more appropriate. Spirulina algae and wild herbs are also alkaline. A smoothy in the morning from ½ cucumber, ¼ red onion, 1 cup of water and 1-2 teaspoons of spirulina flour mixed in a blender awakens your spirits and suppresses your appetite. Now and then, you can also choose the sweet version: Whisk a banana, an apple and 3-4 figs or dates with water. Since the microalgae consist of 60-70% high-quality protein, you don't have to be afraid of muscle atrophy even with a longer spirulina juice cure. Alternatively, treat yourself to an avocado smoothy with wild herbs from traffic-free areas every morning.

Apple cider vinegar cleanses and regenerates the body

For centuries people have used apple cider vinegar for all kinds of health problems. It has anti-inflammatory and antibacterial properties and thus helps fight infections. It is also a typical home remedy for styes. It is also a home remedy for styes. Add two tablespoons of naturally cloudy apple cider vinegar to a glass of hot water, dip a clean cloth in and gently dab the sty.

You don't need to be afraid of acidosis when drinking apple cider vinegar in water. No acidic products build in the metabolism. After energy production, alkaline minerals in particular remain. The same happens with sour apples, lemons, grapefruit or berries.

Apple cider vinegar cleanses, detoxifies, decalcifies and rejuvenates your body inexpensively.

It has a positive effect on metabolism, blood sugar, liver, intestines, blood vessels and skin. Apple cider vinegar also strengthens the immune system and has a stimulating effect. As a true miracle cure, it kills harmful intestinal bacteria and can thus contribute to a healthy intestinal flora. It also relieves typical digestive problems such as flatulence or constipation.

Since apple cider vinegar detoxifies the body, suppresses appetite and boosts fat burning, you can use it as a secret weapon on the way to your dream figure. At least, this is what Hadjer Bouderbala and her Algerian research colleagues demonstrate. In their preliminary study, they searched for new treatments for obesity based on medicinal plants. The scientists gave rats apple cider vinegar and a high-fat diet for 30 days. By comparing it to the control group that did not receive apple cider vinegar, they concluded the following:

The metabolic disorders caused by a high-fat diet thwart by taking apple cider vinegar.

They attested to its satiating, blood fat and blood sugar lowering effect. It can also prevent vascular changes or vascular calcification. (Bouderbala et al., 2016)

Ben Hmad Halima and his fellow Tunisian researchers found that apple cider vinegar supplementation, unlike synthetic antioxidants, mitigates oxidative stress. And with that, it counteracts the "Deadly Quartet". This metabolic syndrome describes the joint occurrence of several symptoms or clinical pictures: obesity, especially in the abdomen, increased fasting blood sugar, lipid levels and high blood pressure. Causes for oxidative stress mainly due to free radicals are environmental influences, bright sunlight, too little sleep or emotional stress.

Halima et al. could confirm the earlier results of their Algerian colleagues (Bouderbala et al. 2016) that apple cider vinegar reduces the risk of obesity. It can, therefore, reduce the risk of obesity-related diseases by preventing lipid metabolism disorders and vascular changes or vascular calcification. (2018)

Apple cider vinegar keeps the gut healthy by helping to remove toxins and waste before they can harm the body. It also promotes digestion, detoxifies the liver, purifies the blood and stimulates the growth of good, beneficial bacteria in the intestines.

Ana CLG Mota and her Brazilian research colleagues evaluated the antifungal activity of apple cider vinegar on candida spp. That is a fungal infection of the deeper tissues. They concluded that apple cider vinegar has antifungal properties against candida spp. It, therefore, represents a possible therapeutic alternative for patients with denture stomatitis or inflammation of the oral mucosa. (2015)

Apple cider vinegar also helps stabilize pH levels, thereby reducing sweat odor. A disturbed pH value in the body can lead to an unpleasant body odor. In addition, mix a teaspoon of apple cider vinegar with a glass of water and essential oils and pour the mixture into a spray bottle. Spray with it. Apply it to the armpits or other affected areas. The unpleasant smell disappears when the apple cider vinegar deodorant dries up. You can also cleanse your skin with apple cider vinegar. Toxins channel out of the body through the skin. On the other hand, essential nutrients absorb through the pores. The vinegar detoxifies and softens the skin.

If you want to reap all of the health benefits of apple cider vinegar, take 1-2 tablespoons in a glass of water half an hour before a meal. If you want to get its full effect, it isbetter to buy raw, unfiltered, organic apple cider vinegar as it contains many essential enzymes. This naturally cloudy, unpasteurized variety with the so-called vinegar mother is even said to help against tinnitus.

Personal experience: Years ago, I drank apple cider vinegar before lunch and lost 6 kg without following a diet. I did not know about its weight-loss effects at the time. I also lost weight during the years of mourning. At the moment, I weigh 58 kg again. For this book project, I have rediscovered apple cider vinegar. That is how I became aware of the connection between apple cider vinegar and weight loss. I will now drink a tablespoon of naturally cloudy apple cider vinegar in a glass of water before breakfast and dinner. Let us see if the scales will show 54 kg again soon.

Cistus detoxifies, strengthens the immune system and is effective against SARS-CoV-2

Cistus (from the Greek kistos), the genus of plants containing about 20 species, forms the family of the cistus plants (Cistaceae). The medicinal tea made from the Cretan cistus is also called gray hairy cistus. Thanks to its antioxidants and polyphenols, the potent medicinal plant strengthens our immune system by protecting the cells from free radicals.

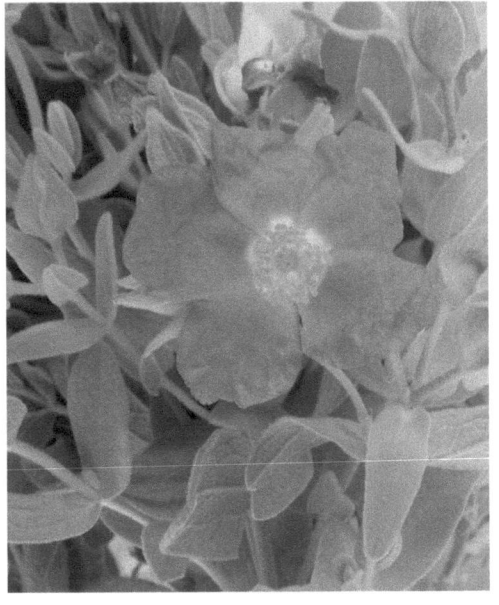

If you drink Cistus tea regularly, you will be safe from colds and flu because the effect against bacteria and viruses is phenomenal.

I can confirm this, and you can also learn this from other users. It also detoxifies the body as its polyphenols bind heavy metals and remove them from the body. Cistus tea also helps with acne and neurodermatitis by dabbing. It even protects the heart far more than red wine, as its polyphenols keep the blood vessels free of deposits and regulate cholesterol levels. (Weidner 2011)

Agnieszka Kuchta and her twelve Polish research colleagues found that the administration of Cistus incanus reduced cardiovascular risk factors such as oxidative stress and dyslipidemia. That speaks all for enjoying Cistus incanus tea daily to prevent atherosclerotic cardiovascular disease. (Kuchta 2019)

Helena Moreira and her four scientific colleagues were able to show that cistus and pomegranate extracts reduce the growth of cancer cells in cancer of the human breast (MCF-7) and colon (LOVO). Their results suggest that the polyphenol-rich extracts tested could be helpful in people exposed to oxidative stress. The use of cistus and pomegranate extracts as a complementary therapy for cancer diseases could also become possible.

According to statements by Saxon Borreliosis self-help groups, taking leaf preparations from Cistus creticus L. (Cistaceae) significantly improved their symptoms. That prompted Hans W. Rauwald and his colleagues from the University of Leipzig and the Fraunhofer Institute for Cell Therapy and Immunology to investigate the definitive anti-Borrelia active ingredients of C. creticus. With the conclusion that the use of C. creticus preparations by self-help groups for Lyme disease can be regarded as a reasonable therapeutic approach. For the first time, isolated epimanoyl oxide and carvacrol could evaluate as the most promising candidates for drug development and to develop labdanum-based phytomedicine, respectively. (Rauwald et al., 2019)

Cistus is currently of particular importance concerning corona. There is a cistus preparation called Cystus 052, which has been tested by the Fraunhofer Institute Leipzig for its effectiveness against the coronavirus since last year. With now sensational results. The extract shows phenomenal effects against bacteria and viruses, in general, and has also tested for its effectiveness against SARS-CoV-2.

I've been drinking cistus tea from time to time for years to detox and strengthen my immune system.

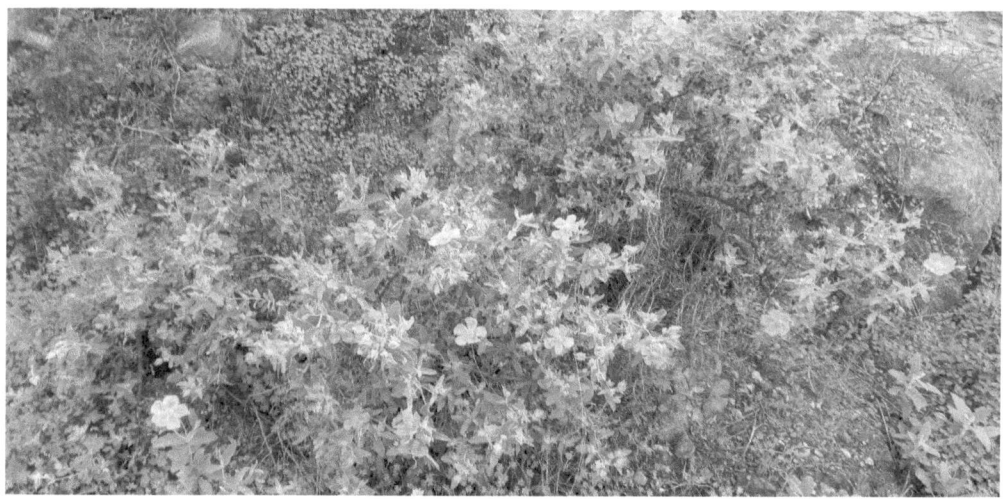

VI. HOW WE STRENGTHEN OUR SOULS AND MINDS

During our recent holiday in the Auvergne, I realized again how easy it is to regenerate internally. We wanted to cool down in France, as the 40+ degrees in the Algarve can sometimes be difficult for an older body. With the baguette and red wine cure (but only one glass a day), I would have thought of constipation or gaining weight. But the opposite was the case. I lost weight and calmed down. The latter was probably because the world calamities left me unaffected by the lack of a TV and PC. When we completely switch off from everyday life, we can regain emotional balance. However, the latter is not always so easy. Thus I propose the following approaches to inner strengthening, which you can also integrate into your daily routine.

How we breathe ourselves healthy and lively

If you have too little oxygen in your body, you become tired and often suffer from pain, ergo inflammation. Most diseases, including cancer, thrive in an oxygen-poor environment. The breath is like the litmus test for the inner state. The more anxious and restless we are, the shorter and shallower our breaths. An optimal oxygen supply for the body is elementary, especially in stressful situations. Deep breathing, therefore, helps against excitement and promotes health and well-being.

Shock, stress or permanent states of anxiety form stress acids in the body, which result in hyperacidity and shallow breathing. So if you want to calm your nerves in today's confusing phase of life that the coronavirus and the war in Europe are forcing us on, you better take a few deep breaths more often during the day.

We've gotten used to breathing shallowly over the past hectic period. Therefore, we take in little oxygen. However, an oxygen-rich environment protects us from germs. Because viruses, bacteria and parasites can hardly exist in it.

Besides our shallow breathing, we wolf down our food and move very little. Thereby, we hardly mobilize our respiratory, circulatory and detoxification systems. It leads to acidosis and a downward spiral for the body and life. The body and mind get tired.

Too little oxygen in the body makes us tired, and we often suffer from pain and inflammation. We need oxygen to supply all cells precisely, the mitochondria, with nutrients and vital substances. These power plants of our cells can thus produce the fuel for our body. Shallow breathing, drinking little and poor posture lead to reduced oxygen intake and hyperacidity.

The best and cheapest way to alkalize the body is deep abdominal breathing and exercise. Or you drink soda water, preferably two hours before eating or before sleeping, two to three hours after your last meal. Because otherwise, it would neutralize the stomach acid needed for digestion.

In yoga, I learned various ways of breathing, mainly how to lengthen the breath. Take your time and make sure the breath flows smoothly and evenly without choking. The so-called 4-7-8 method is also becoming more and more popular: With your mouth closed, breathe in silently through your nose and mentally count to 4. Hold your breath, count to 7 and breathe out through your mouth, counting to 8. You can also do this breathing exercise if you have trouble falling asleep, especially holding your breath. It should better fill the lungs with oxygen, circulating through the whole body. In this way, the organism relaxes and makes it easier to fall asleep.

In addition to this relaxation technique, another breathing exercise to ensure even breathing, a balanced flow of energy and quality sleep is alternating nasal breathing. It has a relaxing effect and helps with colds, exhaustion, depression and headaches. Likely, it should be carried out at least twice a day, also in stressful situations.

1. Sit upright and relax your upper body, neck and head. Breathe in and out slowly, quietly, and in a relaxed manner.
2. Close the left nostril with the ring finger of your right hand and breathe in slowly through the right nostril.
3. Now, close your right nostril with your thumb and exhale completely through the left nostril as slow as possible.
4. Now breathe in slowly through the left nostril again and out through the right. Repeat this breath cycle two more times.

Fear and other trained thought patterns

You wouldn't believe how strong the effect of our trained view of things is. It reflects the strangest symptoms and phenomena. Don't you sometimes fear what might happen in the future? Do you sometimes imagine your death? We are mostly unconsciously trained from childhood on to develop fear. It is done by persistently looking at the next moment, fueled by memories.

I, too, used to be afraid of the future, even though my grandmother Maria, a walking encyclopedia of biblical wisdom, always said: Don't worry about the next day because it will take care of its own. All my deceased loved ones have contacted me in one way or another on the physical plane or shown me their spiritual world. I am looking forward to reuniting with them one day. However, even now, I do not feel separated from them. Because when something crucial happens in my life, they report it regularly. In the last 4-5 years, I experienced this with my late husband, as you can read in the books "Beyond Death" and "Sad News". Since I was quoting my paternal grandmother, here is an experience with her that has to do with the beginning of my writing career:

Grandma Maria came on Thursday, September 3rd, 1998, with her unique smell. She brushed against me as I sat at the computer as if she was standing behind me. She wanted to draw my attention to a special event. Perhaps the page with my interview was rattling through the press at the printing and publishing house. The following morning, my mother called and said: Today, you are the paper's star: an almost one-page interview with a large colour photo of you and your book. I told her about my scent experience. My mother said: That is strange! When I was reading the article, I had the feeling as if she had been looking over my shoulder. (Meyer 2021, p. 65 f.)

So we don't need to be afraid that things won't go on with us once we leave our physical shell. Life is much easier without the tiresome body anyway: no pain, no hunger, no thirst, no exhaustion. So once we leave the *vale of tears*, things get going. Karl Marx was probably aware of this when he said:

Death is not a misfortune for the one who dies but for the one who survives. What other effects do trained thought patterns have? Feelings of guilt, inhibitions, fear of failure, constantly looking for the blame in others, assessing and judging, accepting everything without asserting yourself energetically, avoiding conflicts, always digging in the past, always seeing the negative, but not loving yourself, being able to offer others help again and again, cannot reorganize their own life, cannot pass on love and thus build or maintain partnerships. The good news: You can change your thinking! Simply by recognizing, identifying and raising awareness. In this way we take power from these thought patterns and errors.

Fear of the unknown can trigger panic and shortness of breath

Fear burdens and blocks us. It also prevents us from thinking, acting and making decisions. Fear robs us of our zest for life and often lets us mix the salad of worries in bed for so long that it deprives us of sleep. We usually feel helpless and at the mercy of our fear. I am just reminding you of the worldwide fear that the coronavirus has triggered. The Göttingen anxiety researcher and psychiatrist Prof. Dr Borwin Bandelow believes that fearing the virus and its spread is far from overblown.

www.aerztezeitung.de/Politik/Die-Angst-vor-dem-Coronavirus-ist-weit-ueberzüge-408048.html

I am more afraid of the genetically engineered vaccination than of the disease. This so-called vaccination forces our cells to form a virus or parts of it and is alien to our nature. And, since there are plenty of immune-boosting plants out there, why take chances when we have natural remedies? Especially since Hippocrates, the father of modern medicine, demanded that our food should be our remedy. Have you ever seen syringes grow on trees or sprout from the ground?

Anyway, I hope we'll be over the worst when the book comes out. Lawsuits had been filed already in The Hague. Let us look back at previous pandemics and the number of deaths from other diseases worldwide. We could question whether it is worth driving people's health, social contacts and the entire global and financial economy into a downward spiral. We are always ruled by microorganisms anyway. Gut bacteria control our immune system, which generally copes better with viruses than with the mountains of animal fat that many people gorge on. Degreasing should be the priority instead of inoculating. But that would hinder the socially acceptable death.

Many people become scared and anxious when confronted with a new, supposedly unmanageable threat.

Hundreds of thousands of people die from hospital germs and household accidents. And in the winter of 2017/2018, 25,100 people died from the flu – without panic breaking out, probably due to a lack of media attention.

Dr med. Jens Edrich, like many of his colleagues, says in a video regarding vaccination: It is best to deal with the disease to experience immunological training. This debate is crucial. The corona measures lack reflection.
https://www.youtube.com/watch?v=20inTkjy9dE

Edrich also draws attention to the psychological side. A positive test gives you a fear of the disease that you wouldn't have without it. The fear of the coronavirus can even trigger panic attacks and shortness of breath. Corona quarantine can also lead to anxiety. In another stressful situation, I've had my breath taken away.

Personal experience: a neighbor friend of mine also has prophetic dreams from time to time and told me about a dream in which my late husband Peter had a fatal motorcycle accident. I looked at her in horror, to which she said: Well, he wasn't dead after all. When I woke up the night about three weeks later, Peter and the scooter weren't there. I started hyperventilating. Despite rapid breathing, I had the feeling that I wasn't getting enough air. My fear for Peter competed with my fear of suffocation. I called Csöpi and could hardly speak for lack of the air: Your dream ... Peter ... he's gone ... with the scooter.

When the police were at the front door, I thought of the worst. But Peter only was taken to the hospital with head and knee bruises and missing front teeth.

Singing and laughing strengthen the immune system

Laughter and singing are also medicine against fear. Or, when we feel insecure or afraid, we may hum or whistle to ourselves.

I was already active as a singer in the school choir and later in choirs in different countries. In a study by the University of Frankfurt, Günter Kreutz and his colleagues were able to show that singing in a choir, but not just listening, has a positive effect on secretory immunoglobulin A, cortisol and the emotional state. Researchers from the Frankfurt Institute for Music Education studied together with the Institute for Psychology and the German Singers Association. They tested the hypothesis: Musical activities influence subjective moods and physiological processes in the autonomic nervous systems of amateur choir members of a Frankfurt church community. They rehearsed Mozart's Requiem for a performance. Next to subjective surveys, the researchers measured the cortisol and immunoglobin A levels. The results showed notable positive changes in immune competence of the singers but not in the listeners to choral music. So, let us sing happily, which will also activate your pineal gland!

It would be desirable if health insurance contributions would be not only negatively influenced by illnesses in future health care reforms. It would be fairer if singing activities in amateur choirs and other initiatives that strengthen the immune system could also evaluate. If you give something to the community, you could get something in return.

I was born with a weak immune system. As a six-week-old baby, I suffered from an inflammation of the lungs and later of the pleura. After two surgeries at the age of 3 and 5, Prof. Wolfgang Jäger in Heidelberg pricked my old age cataract at age 13. That is why I am taking the immune boosters from A to Z alternately as a kind of second immune system. And using the breathing exercises shown in Part III and other spiritual and mental strengthening agents and preparing the dishes from my healthy kitchen from page 79 on daily or create new ones.

The memory of our ancestors as a source of strength

Many people use set rituals to reflect, commemorate their loved ones and deal with death. They need orientation and support. Therefore, they like to fall back on religious rites and ceremonies when they become aware of their limits. Or when they confront unexplainable or uncontrollable. On the November memorial days, a modern man may feel compelled to visit the cemetery to attune himself to the calm and peace of the dead. It's different for me. I think almost daily of one or the other of my loved ones who are no longer in their bodies. I also experience a lot with them that others cannot explain. The reason is that most of my mother's relatives have or had experience with the spirit world. Through lively exchange with the family and other people who experience supernatural things, I have opened up the so-called inexplicable in various ways. The experience with my father, who died twenty-four years ago, and my husband, who left his body five years ago, shaped me mostly. You can find out more about these contacts in the above-mentioned memorial books.

In my life, telepathy, daily and nightly prophetic visions, past life regressions, automatic writing and painting were more or less part of everyday life. I experienced the latter when I needed a quick birthday present for my brother-in-law. And in just under three minutes, I drew the tree that adorns the cover of my novel Family Code. I originally wrote this book for my relative Doris Day. So she could learn how her German family members lived during the two world wars, in the 1950s and into the new millennium. At the tree, you could perhaps say, well, she had a creative phase there. But what does the following video by Antonio Gasparetto, which lets the old masters work through him, tell you? Who, as a trans- medium, gives them his hands, sometimes also his feet, so that they can channel their works through him:

www.youtube.com/watch?v=URM8KGpjztE

When people tell me we only live once, and after death everything ends, I reply, better not count on it. Perhaps you will change your mind when you watch the video of Luiz Antonio Gasparetto. He, in a trance, paints originals by deceased painters at breakneck speed, without looking at the canvas or at the colours he is choosing. Dwellers in spiritual dimensions use mediums to tell us: look, we still exist! Again and again, they try to contact their loved ones in the flesh. But how do most people react? With ignorance. Or they only say: Oh, why is the light flashing all the time on the anniversary of my husband's death? Or: What are those strange letters in the TV grit? Many people consider such phenomena to be coincidental. And few think of ghosts when something inexplicable happens. Or they say it was a ghost but rarely dig deeper. But when we die one day and return home to the world vibrating with higher frequencies, we will be happy if our loved ones recognize our efforts to make contact and are happy to let us fulfill their wishes. For example, I had wanted a pingpong table for a long time and asked Maurits to look out for it or build one. He said spontaneously, better buy one used in France. In the first week of our vacation, we visited the largest second-hand shop near our town. By entering, a blue ping-pong table just came in for about an eighth of the new price. Coincidence? Couldn't it be that the universe (perhaps my late husband) telepathically or in a dream prompted the owner of said ping-pong table to donate his unused, space-consuming table to charity?

Whenever something wondrous happens, I think of requests from the spiritual world. Gifted and less gifted spirit painters also work via water crystal photography, which I present in Water Crystals: Message of the Souls and my earlier water books. There, water is the medium of communication, as in homeopathy, by the way. In my book Healthy without Drugs, I inform about another project of the spiritual world: the scalar wave analysis. At this, we do not need lengthy and expensive diagnostic measures such as allergy tests, hair analyses, blood, urine, stool and other examinations. See page 56 ff.

Through the cooperation with a German naturopath and a Portuguese health practitioner, I convinced myself in several tests with different people over two years that the scalar wave analysis shows about two hundred correct parameters in less than two minutes. The scalar wave analysis and therapy are ridiculed by the disease industry's trolls, because they cannot work according to the traditional understanding of physics. But the values were confirmed, among other things, by blood and hair analyses in German and Portuguese laboratories. I think this simple type of diagnostics and therapy is another gift from the spiritual world to make life easier for us in the earthly vale of tears.

Is there a guarantee for a happy life?

What do you want from life? Most of my readers will probably say, live healthy and happy in peace and prosperity. But many do nothing at all for their health. They argue about trifles and spend their money on short-term gratifications. Often they work in a job that doesn't challenge them and doesn't give room for their talents and passions. Or they get bogged down in an office, although they would prefer to be in the fresh air and would then be happier even with the garbage disposal.

If you feel caught and say yes, but I have to pay my rent and two kids to feed, how am I supposed to work something I enjoy but doesn't pay my bills. I can only recommend that you ask the world leader, the universe or your loved ones in the afterlife for what you want. Or you could deal with what you are striving for in your free time. It was the same for me. I just started writing travelogues. After that, everything came to me by itself:

Health expert Halima Neumann visited me in California and asked if I could translate her acidosis book. That would be good training for my doctoral thesis in nutritional science. When I returned to Germany, Barbara Simonsohn got in touch with me. She heard about the translation and asked if I would translate her Papaya book. Since I mentioned my dissertation on the blue-green alga and the immune system, Barbara informed Mrs Jünemann from Windpferd-Verlag. So it happened that I was able to introduce the beneficial blue-green microalgae with my best-seller *Spirulina, das blaugrüne Wunder* in German-speaking and Eastern European countries.

If you are not quite sure what you want, it is best to make a wish list and write down ten wishes. Read through them daily and add new wishes for each fulfilled one. Dealing with your desires will crystallize all by itself. The more you go into detail about what you want, the better.

Healing thoughts help the immune system

Just like diet and exercise, the way you think affects your health. But it is not enough if you think positively in the spirit of "Everything will be fine". You only give your thoughts strength when you connect them with intense emotions and have your goal in your mind's eye, just as you will achieve it would.

With the help of the mind, we can influence our physical and mental health. Studies show: that there is a constant dialogue between the brain and the immune system. To do this, they use messengers, which couple to the receptors on the cell membrane surfaces. Our moods, attitudes, and thoughts impact what chemical messages (neurotransmitters or neuropeptides) are sent and how they are received. According to Dr David L. Felten, Professor of Neurobiology and Anatomy, the immune system connects to the nervous system in addition to neuropeptides. Nerve fibres reach all the organs of the immune system and establish direct contact with the immune cells. www.researchgate.net/scientific-contributions/David-L-Felten-38152313

How we react to everyday life, stressful situations and negative news affect the immune system efficacy. People who are cynical, hostile or suppress anger are more likely to have heart attacks and atherosclerosis. Especially in times of Corona, negative news is scary. And every kind of fear and every negative feeling automatically triggers a stress response in the body. When you experience negative situations, you usually feel it in your breathing, which virtually stops. Avoid negative influences with positive thoughts. And with a smile. Even if you fake a laugh, the pituitary gland releases endorphins. You also generate happiness hormones when you breathe consciously and think that every breath cheers you up and strengthens your immune system.

VII. STAYING BEAUTIFUL EVEN IN LOOKDOWN TIMES

We could all see it during the lockdown period: Some people came across as a bit unique without going to the hairdresser. As an incurable autodidact, it is important to me to initiate you into the art of improvisation. I not only cut my loved ones and my hair. Once, I even made my mother's frayed, self-pierced ear-piercing ready for use again. At that time, I worked for a doctor and had easy access to all the necessary utensils: sterilized anesthetic syringe, scalpel, curved needle and thread. I found out from my hiking companion that her husband, an American, sews up his cuts himself with a regular needle and thread!

Homemade haircut and hair wave creations

If you need a haircut or perm, you can employ a trick that I took on for half a century. In this respect, you can look forward to another lockdown with ease. If you want to cut your hair, wash it as usual. Then, using a tail comb, pick up a strand and trim the tip. Or as much as you like. Then take a hair roller and wind up this strand. Now continue doing this with the next strand until all the hair is cut and twisted.

You might want to cut off your long straight hair as I did at age 23 when I pulled a Marsha Hunt memorial Afro. For it, you either use very small, preferably self-adhesive curlers, especially if you want curls that will not show a perm. Otherwise, you can use the especially thin perm curlers. I currently use the tiniest self-adhesive rollers alternated with the most-largest perm rollers.

Daily facial gymnastics with muscle training

There is nothing good unless you do it. With this shortest poem, Erich Kästner wanted to express: We must fight for human rights. Just as consistently, we jump at the opportunity to achieve what we want. Not as a New Year's resolution that we will have forgotten in mid-January. Many of the holistic beauticians and naturopaths I interviewed 15 years ago for a book advise their clients to do the following exercises. Do each of the following exercises for a maximum of 90 seconds. Squeeze each muscle for 6 seconds and pause for 4 seconds.

Exercise 1

Stand or sit straight, shoulders down, backwards. Bring your shoulder blades together, hold for 6 seconds, then sit up straight. Squeeze your neck muscles and resist with your hands.

Exercise 2

Against the double chin: Press against the chin with the thumbs and hold against it with the palate muscle. See also Exercise 7.

Exercise 3

Massage the muscles in the front and behind the ear. Push the ear forward with the index or middle finger and hold against it with the ear muscle. Pull the ear upwards and hold against it with the upper ear muscle. Ditto backwards. This exercise can even reduce your tinnitus.

Exercise 4

Press the eyebrows up with your fingertips and hold against them with the superior orbicular muscle. Hold your cheekbones under your eyes with your fingers, look up and lift your lower lid. By the way: eyebrow acupressure and drinking hot green or black tea is also an alternative treatment/prevention option for glaucoma.

Exercise 5

Use your fingers to stretch the region above the nose. Counter it with the muscle. Fix your forehead with your fingertips and move the top of your skull.

Exercise 6

Against upper lip lines: Stretch the area above the upper lip outwards and press the lips firmly together for 6-10 seconds. Consistent smoothing of the upper lip area: repeat the above 10-20 times in row 2-3 times a day. You can achieve the same effect if you put a cork between your lips and press firmly.

Exercise 7

One more exercise fighting double chins: Extend your tongue far out and down, hold it for a while, and pull it back out. Repeat this exercise several times; also 3-5 times with tongue curled. Push the lower jaw far forward and up, tense for 6 seconds, and release. Repeat 7-9 times.

When you do the exercises for the first time, you can treat yourself to soreness. Tip: before every workout, take 3-4 spirulina pellets with a glass of water or drink a fruit or vegetable shake with a teaspoon of spirulina flour. Many competitive athletes know that their muscles regenerate faster with spirulina before training.

Cellulite: No more bumps

More and more people are acidic because they neglect the bases. I just saw another family at lunch with pancakes. And that's about it: neither salad nor vegetables or soup to buffer the acids with alkalines. Also, many people only eat pasta with ketchup or mayonnaise. That's one of the reasons teenagers sometimes have ugly dents on their thighs, even those who do competitive sports. The cause is usually an over-acidification of the organism.

Therefore, the bases are also the basis of the treatment for cellulite: lots of greens! As I mentioned before, the root of all evil lies in the acid-forming diet, such as animal protein, sugar, coffee, cola and other soda drinks. Bread, rice and pasta also metabolize acidic like most grains. Athletes mainly eat such concentrated carbohydrates. In addition, stress, anger and worries form acids. High-performance sports and other heavy physical exertion lead to the formation of lactic acid in the body. Our organism reacts to this with increased water retention.

To protect himself, he dilutes the excess acids. In addition, it buffers them with alkaline salts and forms waste dumps, which often show up as unsightly bumps. He extracts these minerals from the bones, the cartilage, the scalp and the veins. So don't be surprised if you don't need a comb anymore, not only in old age. Hair loss, vascular diseases, tooth decay, and osteoporosis are signs of an acidic environment. The acids are partly excreted, partly deposited as waste: in the filter of the connective tissue, on joints, vessel walls and in the excretory organs. So if you suffer from kidney, gallbladder or bladder problems, you should increase the bases instead of eating spaghetti.

If you eat a balanced diet, drink enough water, work out 15 minutes every day and still have cellulite on your thighs, the first thing to do is get your acid-base balance in order. That way, all metabolic processes work smoothly. Besides electrolyte, water and oxygen balance, the acid-base balance is one of the most crucial regulatory systems in our body. It helps maintain blood functions and activates enzymes, friendly bacteria and hormones. That means eating lots of fruit and vegetables, drinking lots of water and avoiding concentrated carbohydrates. That is because they deprive the body of water. That does not mean you can never eat hamburgers, spaghetti, or pizza again. Only the amount of the glue diet is problematic.

Many have the feeling that they eat health-consciously. But they are still acidic, flabby and have a harmed fascia.

By the way, spirulina helps break down acids when under stress. Since the microalga contain all B (stress) vitamins and minerals. So, the best way to reduce cellulite is to eat better, cut your intake of toxins and do a lot of exercises. And a body brush helps as well to smoothen and repair the damaged fascia.

We can delay the aging process

Why do we age at all? As we get older, our cells divide more slowly – the metabolism slows down. External factors can also contribute to rapid aging, such as aggressive oxygen atoms destroying healthy cells in the body. These so-called free radicals are responsible for age spots and are comparable to rust on a car. The skin becomes sallow and wrinkled.

If we walk briskly for just half an hour a day and eat a diet rich in vitamins and minerals, we can achieve a lot. But in today's chemical-radiological environment, it is vital to provide the body with dietary supplements that protect us from oxidative stress as free-radical scavengers. However, we should not take uncontrolled essential substances but rather have our levels tested regularly. Too much selenium can, e. g., lead to gastrointestinal or vision and memory problems and is noticeable by a garlic smell in the breath.

Health and beauty are like retirement planning. If you don't start investing early, you won't have much left. We can compare caring for the body with tending. All sins are stored: sooner or later, the organism or the vehicle owner will receive the receipt. Since my late husband and I were classic automobile dealers in California, we saw a lot of scrapped rust buckets. But if such a classic car is regularly cared for and protected from the sun and salt, it can still drive and shine like on the first day. Speaking of which: I was able to deal with the grief for my husband, who died suddenly, through the books Beyond Death and Sad News, which he wrote with me posthumously and gave a lot of input. As my clairvoyant friend said, Peter would like to write a book with me about the car dealership days in Frankfurt and LA. But my pineal gland probably needs to be stimulated a little more first. That may sound strange to some of my readers. But many widows and widowers have contact with their loved ones in the afterlife. This time was greatly difficult for me after 44 years together. But at moments when I felt Peter's presence were also exhilarating. Like on his brother's birthday. Perhaps Peter's grandnephew, who was three and a half years old, sensed his presence when he spontaneously grabbed my cell phone and took a photo of me. Had Peter even instructed him to do so? Who knows all the secrets of the little ones?

At this age, many children have contact with relatives in the afterlife. But when they share their experiences, parents often think it's their imagination. And they try to suppress such comments from their young children because they do not want them to become public. I figured it out because Moritz and Jonas, my brother's grandsons, had contact with various deceased relatives at that age.

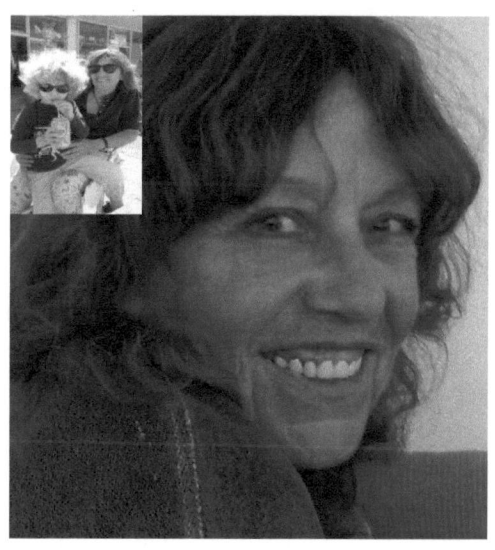

Anyway, Joshua snapped me on Peter's brother's birthday six weeks after his great-uncle, Peter, left his physical shell. As for happiness from spirit life, as you can see from this photo, I don't exactly look like a grieving 68-year-old widow.

By the way, someone asked me recently if I suffer from a gum problem. But I can still bite hard into a Granny Smith without leaving a trace of blood. All my life, have I shown a lot of gums when I laugh. But since it's healthy when your ears are visited, and I don't want to give up laughing under any circumstances, my counterparts and you, my dear readers, will have to get used to this look.

But back to the possible delay in the aging process: Of course, this also has to do with care. The main thing is to prevent acid build-up. Stress, worries, lack of sleep, too much sun, smoking, alcohol, and poor nutrition result in a lack of vital substances and too little exercise stored in the cell water. The latter turns sour over time. Regular training is just as necessary as a healthy diet, around 30 ml of water per kg of body weight every day, enough rest, sleep, fresh air and sun. However, too much exercise, such as extreme physical work or high-performance sports, is counterproductive and creates stress acidity. It would be so easy to give your body what it needs if there wasn't always a weaker self lurking around.

But your body doesn't need an immune dumping vaccine! Because all vaccines contain many toxins. Vaccinators are happy to hide from you that patients who test positive and come to the hospital to give birth or to have their broken leg splinted are immediately transferred to the corona ward, even if they have no symptoms. So now I'm advising those giving birth to have a home birth with a midwife. We hear about such practices from whistleblower support staff. Also, vaccinators don't tell you that twice-vaccinated people are more contagious than unvaccinated people. And how is the latter minority treated? I can only encourage you to write everything down. Since then, millions of videos of doctors, lawyers and journalists questioning government actions have been deleted. The pro-government media's distorted reports are full of lies. Critical scientists are losing their jobs. Judges who pass judgments that are not in line with the government must endure house searches. And opponents of vaccination are described as "dangerous social pests"! Are we there again? Haven't we learned anything from the past?

If you're asking why I keep talking about the disease industry and avoid doctor's offices, let me point you to Western medical history. The award-winning Doctor of Medicine Gerd Reuther assured this in his book *Heilung Nebensache*. His core theses are that there is no healing without self-healing and that the medical systems were and are primarily oriented towards profit, not towards health. Here is an interview in German: https://www.youtube.com/watch?v=OBPK1SaKowk

The following Interview informs about a crucial initiative for the good of humanity: youtube.com/watch?v=SXS-rdu07QI&list=PLTwoZMZdoo7bhFhvbR4tLcSkk6uSCNG-n&index=31

VI. RECIPES FROM DR MEYER'S TIMELY HEALTHY CUISINE

People have less and less time these days for cooking. Therefore you can prepare the following recipes for two persons in just over 30 minutes. Most dishes more quickly.

Teaspoon	tsp
Tablespoon	tbsp
Cup	
Drop	dr
Small	sm
Large	lg
Pinch	pin

Antipasti platter with olive paste

1 cup black olives   mash with
2 cloves of garlic   and
3 tbsp olive oil   fry
Zucchini slices, pieces of pepper and
2 quartered shallots   in a little olive oil; sprinkle with
1 tsp Italian herbs   serve with the olive paste in the middle,
                              pepper from the mill and spelt buns. See page 97.

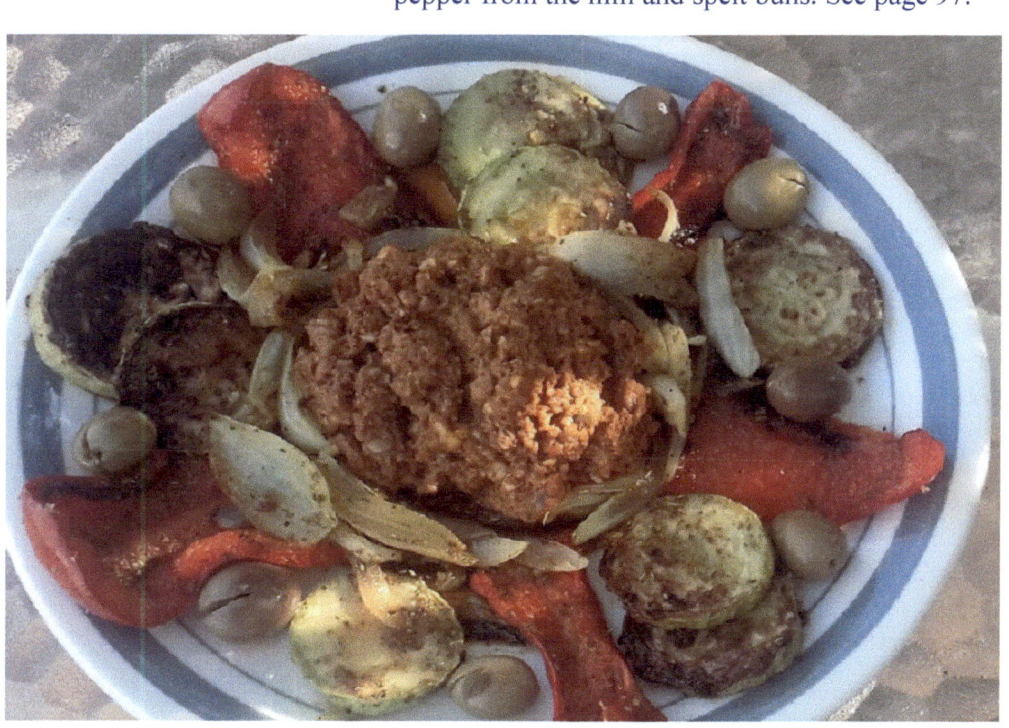

79

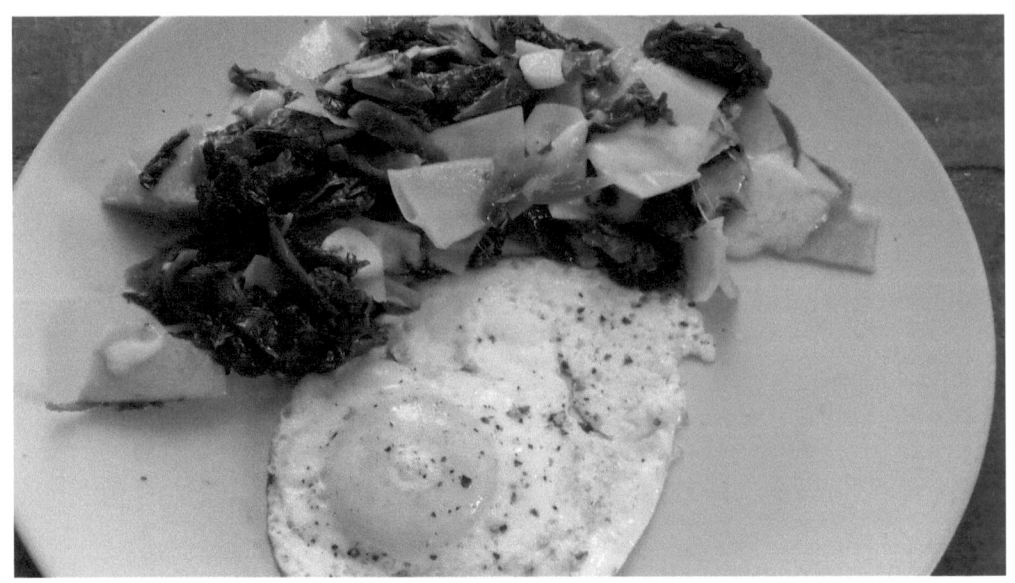

Butter squash with spinach & fried egg

1 red onion	remove the outer skin, quarter, cut length-ways; sautée in
3 tbsp olive oil and	
a pinch of salt	peel and finely chop
3 garlic cloves	add
250 g pumpkin,	peel and slice into slices with a vegetable slicer; wash
2 cups spinach leaves	and put them in a pot or pan; fry
1 or 2 eggs	serve with 1pinch salt and pepper from the mill

Crepe Marianne (vegan)

1 cup spelt flour (630)	or whole grain mix with
1 level tsp baking soda	and
1 pinch Himalayan salt	add
1 tbsp spelt, oat or	almond milk and
½ cup water	mix everything with a whisk stir well, fry in a large, flat
	pan with well-heated
4-6 tbsp of rapeseed oil	

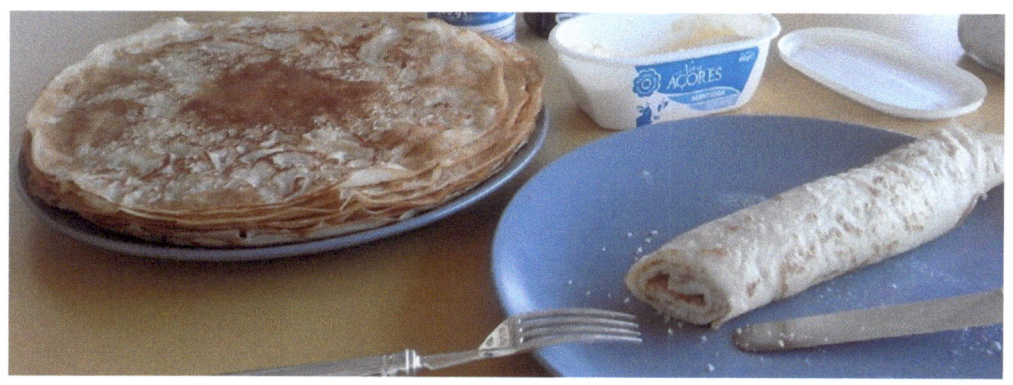

Spelt rolls with pumpkin seeds

500 g spelt flour   mix well with
1 tsp Himalayan salt
2 tsp baking soda   and
4 tbsp organic vinegar from apples and water form balls, dip them in pumpkin seeds and bake at 160° for 25 minutes

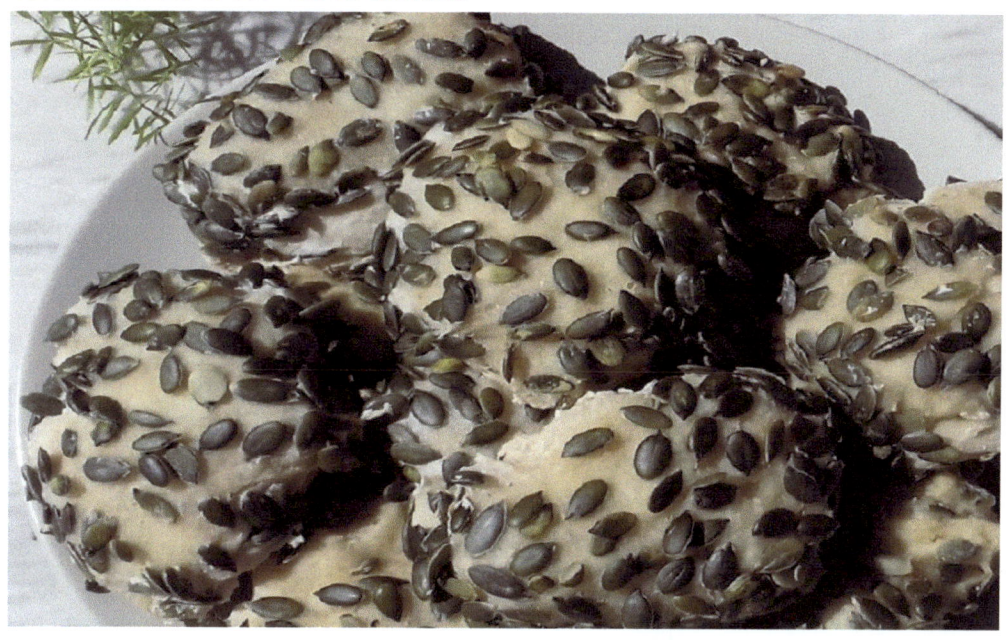

Peas with sweet potatoes

	sautée
1-2 onions	with
3 tbsp of olive	or rapeseed oil in a pan over low heat; slice and add
3 cloves of garlic	peel and cut
1 lg sweet potato	in slices and add along with 3 tbsp of water; after 5 mins add
1 cup of frozen peas	and steam for another 2 minutes, serve one trout per person; see page 90

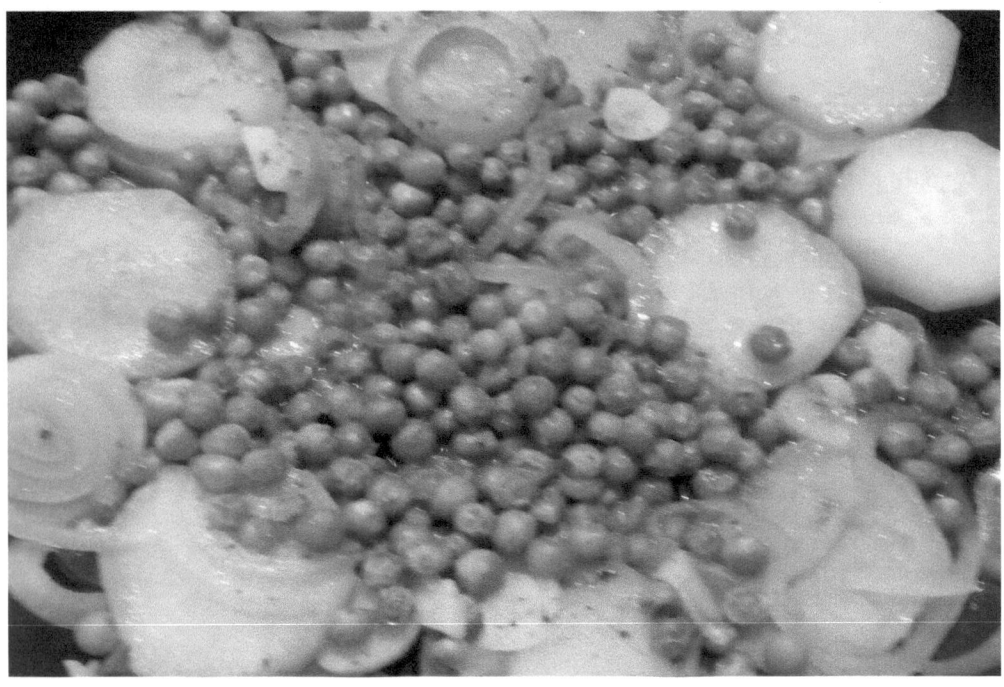

Cream cheese salad with spelt flatbread

1½ cups spelt flour	mix with
½ tsp Himalayan salt	and as much
water	that you get a liquid dough; bake 4 chapatis in a pan
½ head of romaine lettuce	plucked finely, mix with
100 g fresh goat cheese	
2-3 mushrooms	sliced

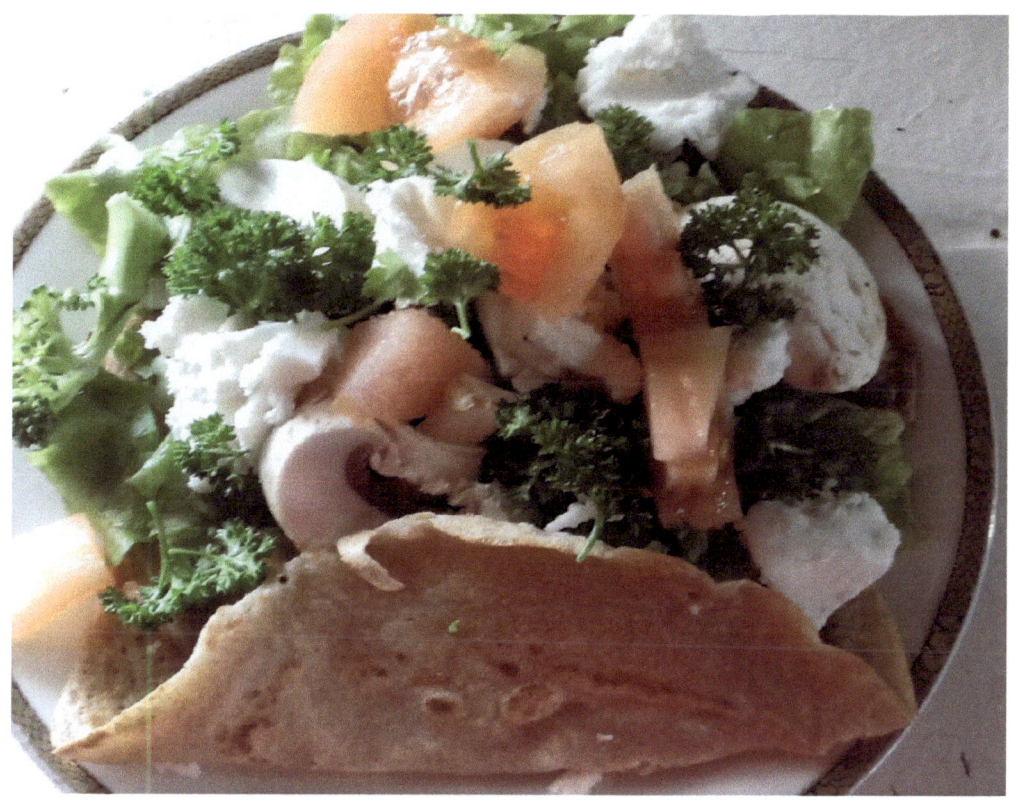

1 tomato	cut into small pieces
3 sprigs of parsley	and
2 tbsp of olive oil	or linseed oil and season as desired; of course, you can also choose any other salad

Fresh veggie-quark

250 g low-fat quark	mixed with
3-4 tbsp of linseed oil	and
250 g seasonal veggies	cut into small pieces

depending on your taste, you can season with a little salt, pepper, basil, parsley, turmeric, ginger or mint to taste; serve with baguette; you can use seasonal fruit with honey instead of vegetables

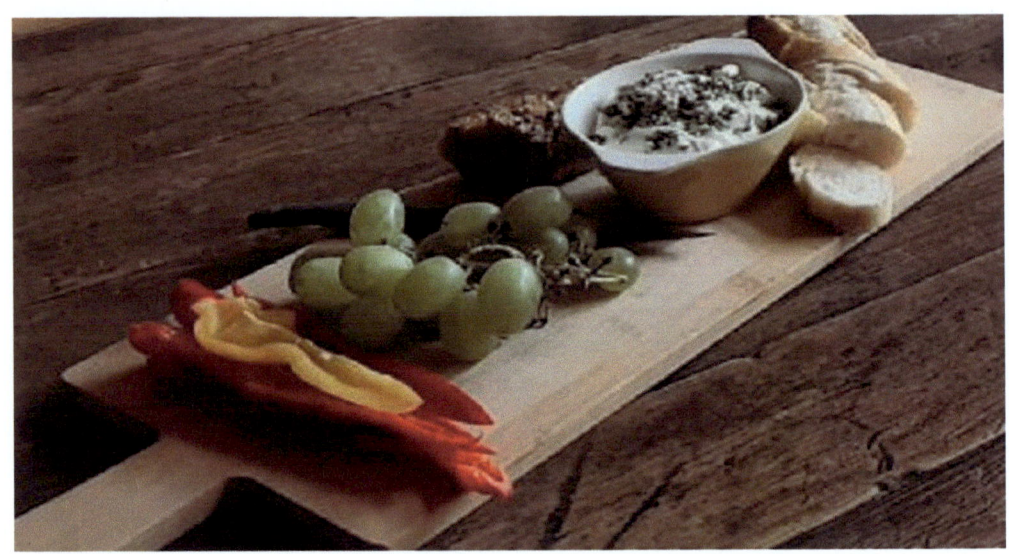

Vegetable cake

2 cups spelt flour	mix with
1 tsp salt	and
1 tsp of baking powder	
1 tbsp flaxseed	soaked in 4 tbsp water
3 tbsp olive oil	and
5 tbsp almond milk	alternatively coconut or oat milk and process into a smooth dough; sautée
250 g mixed vegetables	of your choice and
1-2 onions	in
3 tbsp of olive oil	after cooling thicken with
4 tbsp ground flaxseed	soaked in ½ cup water; mix
200 g sour cream	or sour cream made from almonds, lemon and coconut oil and
200 g organic yogurt	alternatively vegan yogurt with
1 tbsp cornstarch	or 1 tsp psyllium husk powder and
salt & pepper	roll out the dough into a round sheet; grease the bottom and edge of the ring mold with
3 tbsp olive/coconut oil	and line with the dough; bake at 170 °C approx. 30

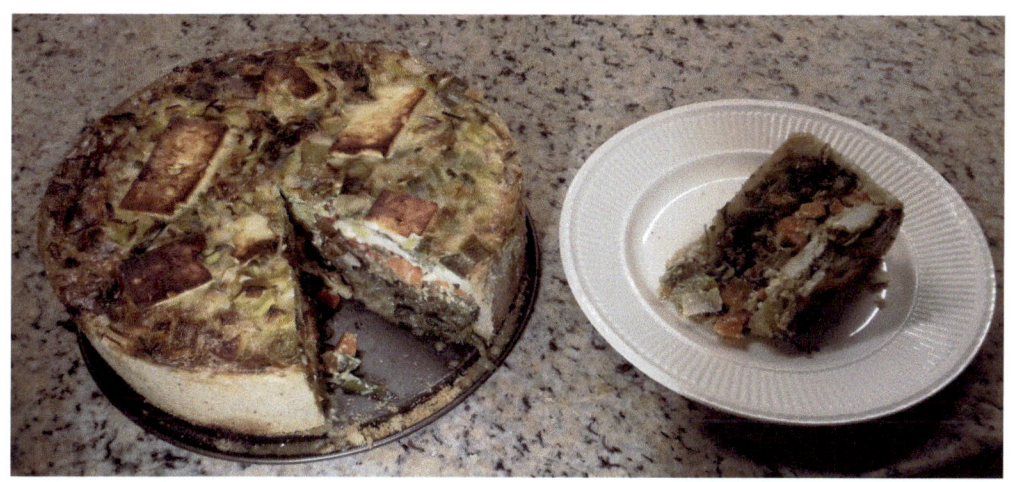

Vegetable pan with mushrooms and sweet potatoes

1-2 onions	sautée with
3 tbsp of olive oil	or rapeseed oil, i.e. let it turn yellow; add
2-3 cloves of garlic	or sliced ginger; brush
1 lg sweet potato	and add it in slices with the skin on; wash and cut
5-6 mushrooms	
1 tomato & 50 g rucola	alternatively chop spinach, cook with 3-4 tbsp water for 8 minutes on a low flame

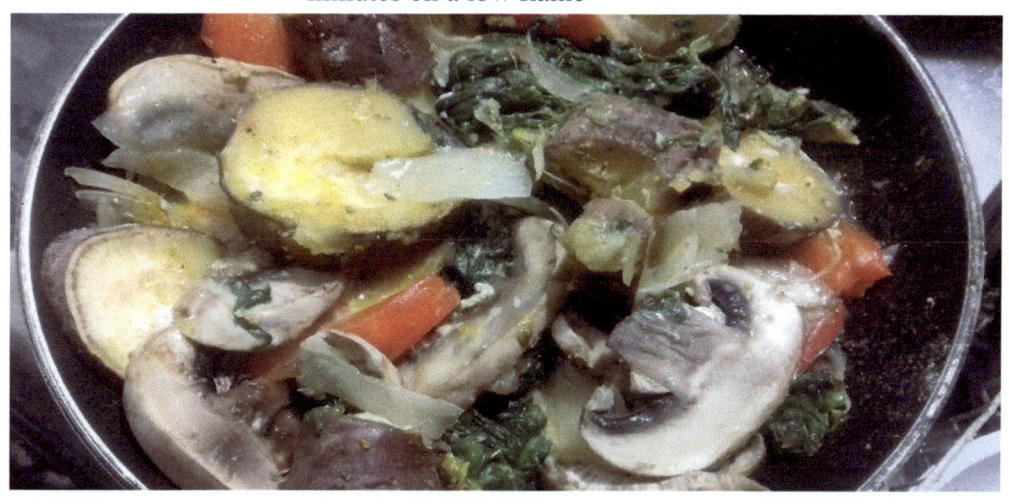

85

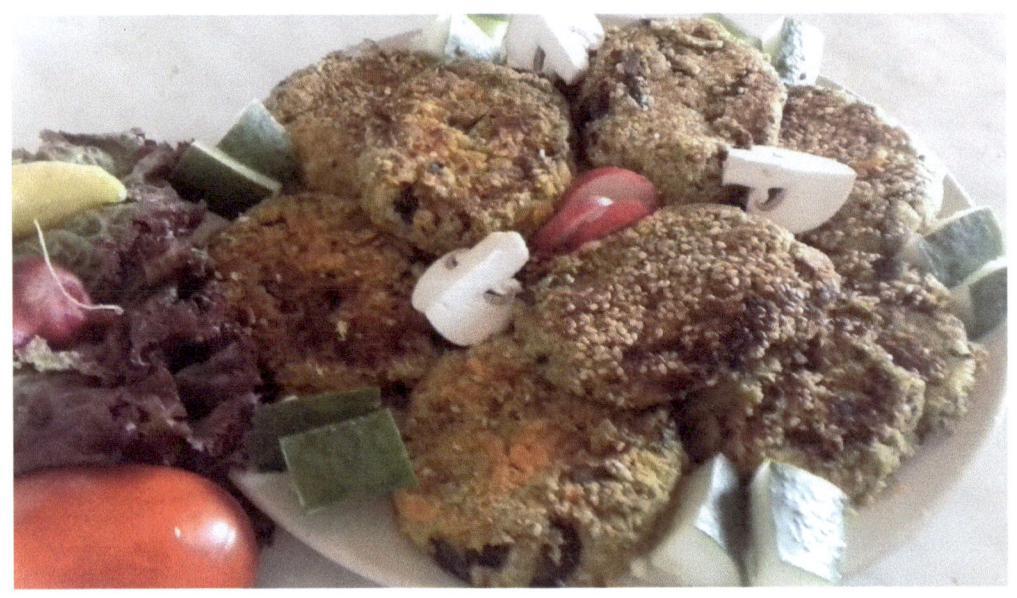

Guacamole with cottage cheese

2 ripe avocados   mash in a bowl with a fork; fold in
200 g of cottage cheese stir in the juice of

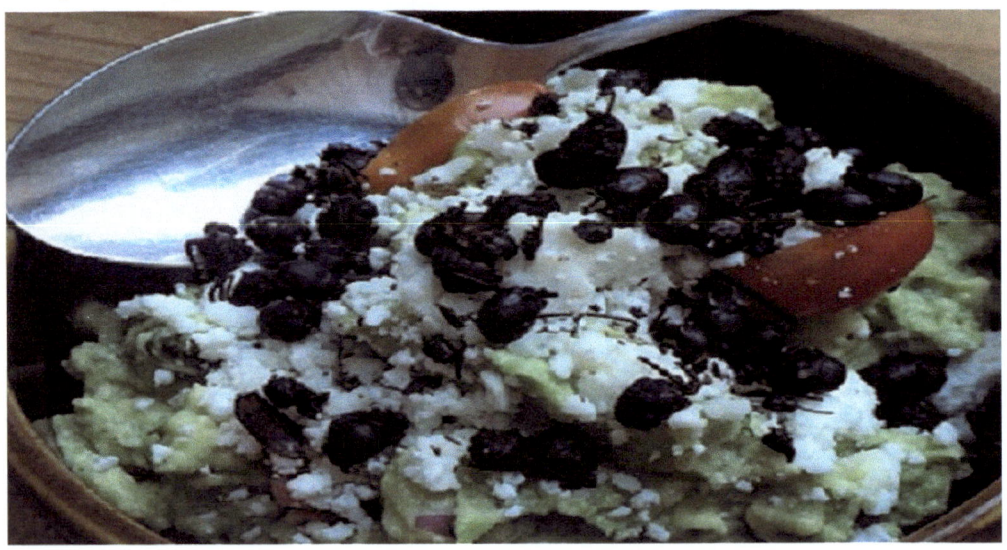

2 cloves of garlic (grated, pressed or very finely chopped) and
¼ tsp cayenne pepper cut
1 tomato into small pieces and spread together with
 ½ teaspoon black olives over the guacamole; along with it are tasty organic corn nachos sometimes bought ones too

Chickpea Meatball

1 tsp chickpeas (canned)	mix with
2 tbsp of flax-seed	in ½ cup water for 15 minutes along with
2 tbsp olive oil	
1 red onion in eighths	
1 tsp mustard	or mustard powder; each
½ tsp ginger, coriander,	
turmeric & curry powder	and puree
8 black olives in a blender add	
2 grated carrots	mix the whole mass with 2 tbsp spelt or oat flour; season with herbs, sea or Himalayan salt and pepper to

taste; form patties; as you wish, you can roll in sesame seeds on both sides and fry them in oil

Cabbage rolls with soy granules

4 tbsp soy granules	soak in
1 cup vegetable broth	(1 vegetable stock cube or 1 tsp grained broth)
1 tbsp flaxseed	
4 tbsp soy sauce	
1 red onion finely diced	
1 tsp mustard powder	
¼ tsp cayenne pepper	and
2 tbsp of olive oil	for 10 minutes; meanwhile cook the leaves
½ white/savoy cabbage	in boiling water for 6-8 minutes; spread little heaps of soy dough on the cabbage leaves, roll them up and secure

with a toothpick; bake with cheese sprinkled on top at 180° for approximately 20 minutes

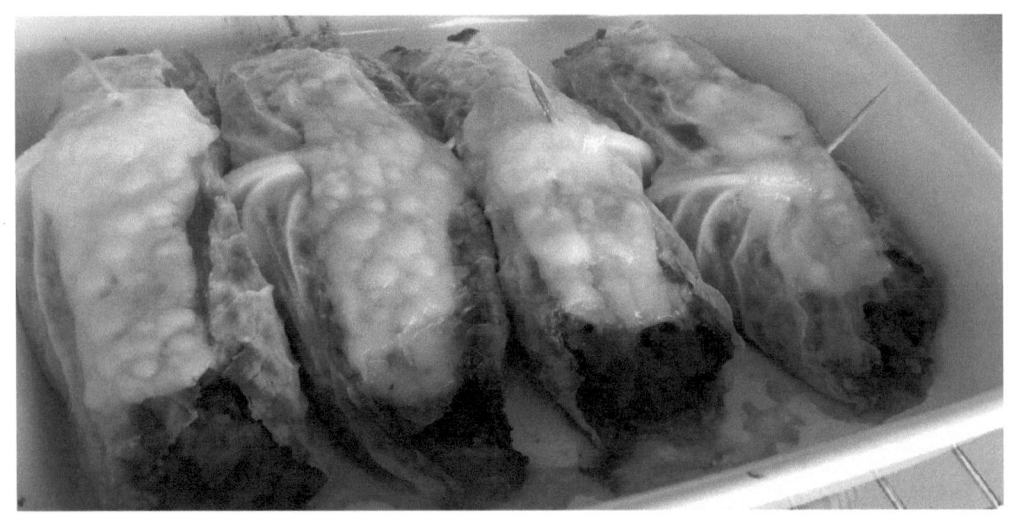

Cabbage and goat cheese meatballs

2 tbsp of flaxseed	soak in ½ cup of water; scrape a
½ pointed cabbage	peel and grate
1 red onion	crumble
100 g goat feta	prepare
½ cup olives	
2 tbsp oat flour	

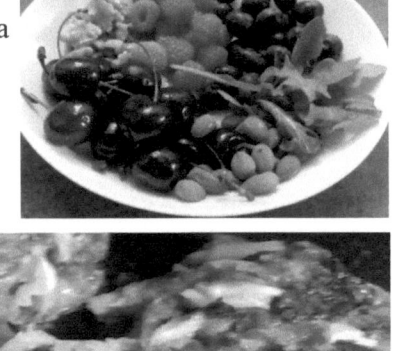

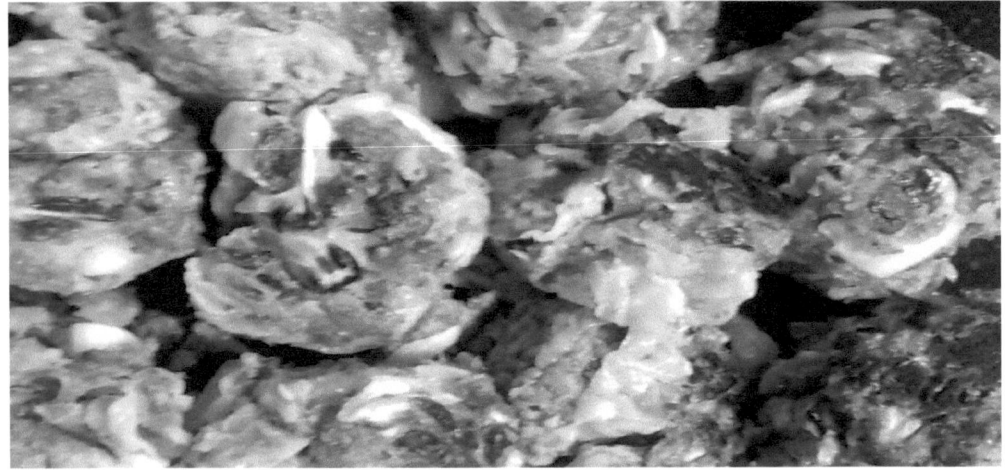

4 tbsp olive or canola oil	and
1 pin cayenne pepper	with the flax-seed and all ingredients to a dough; form patties and brown each side for 3 minutes

By the way: Before every cooked meal, I eat either a fresh food salad or just a few berries and nuts. The food enzymes relieve the pancreas in its function of producing digestive enzymes; cooking food destroys enzymes

Salmon fillet with chicory

2 pieces of salmon fillet	salt lightly, fry in a pan with
3 tbsp olive or canola oil	peel 4 little or 2 large
chicory pods	peel and cut
2 sweet potatoes	simmer for 8 minutes in boiling water; season with
ginger and pepper	from the mill or herbs of your choice

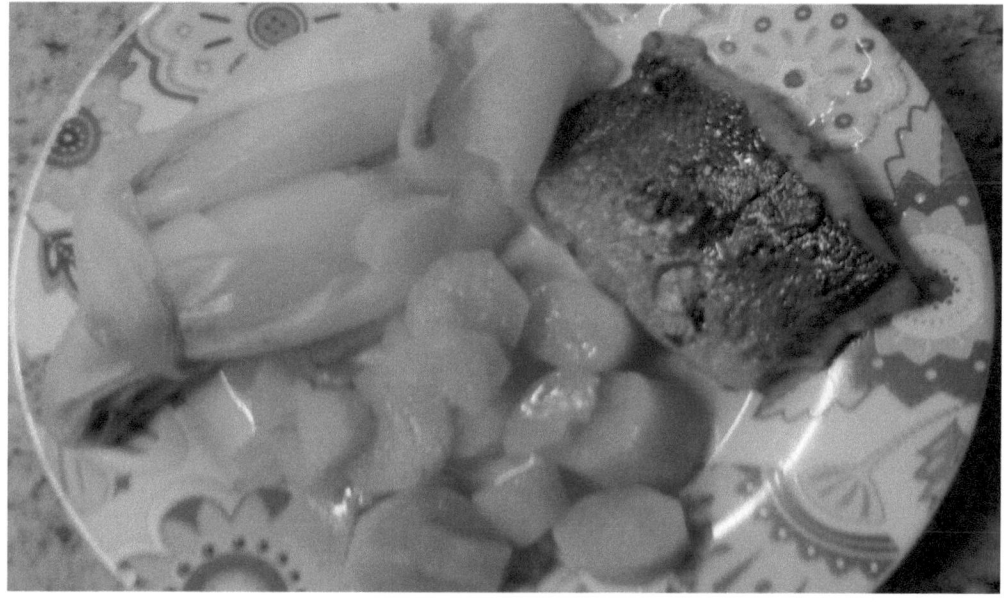

People often ask me why I eat so much salmon. I eat fish two times a week. Mostly wild Alaskan salmon, herring or sardines (they eat plankton). Astaxanthin is considered a powerful antioxidant. Salmon farmers feed the red algae Haematococcus Pluvialis to give the fish a beautiful red color. I prefer to eat salmon instead of just taking astaxanthin capsules.

Trout with chicory

2 trouts	wash, pat dry, salt lightly and brown for 2 minutes each side in
3 tbsp olive oil	and a little water or white wine; add
2 chicory pods	and simmer for 10 minutes, season to taste, spread sliced
80 g goat cheese	over the chicory

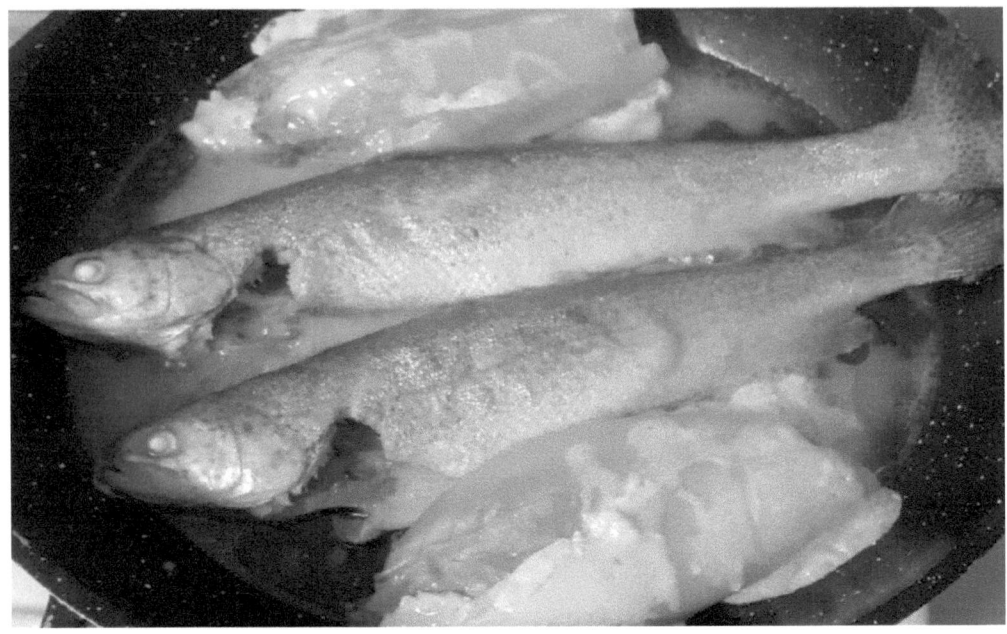

Swiss chard, pumpkin & cheese rolls

1 onion	slice and sauté; add
2 crushed garlic cloves	clean and add
150 g chard	peel
150 g pumpkin	and add it in slices; simmer for 8 minutes
	for the bun dough work up
2 cups spelt flour (630)	with
1 tsp Himalayan salt	
1 tsp baking soda	with 1 cup water to a dough, form balls; dip them in
100 g of crumbly cheese	and place them on a baking tray or in a deep pan with lid
	and bake for approx. 25 minutes at 150° or on a low flame;

you can also put garlic slices on top or add grated garlic to the dough

90

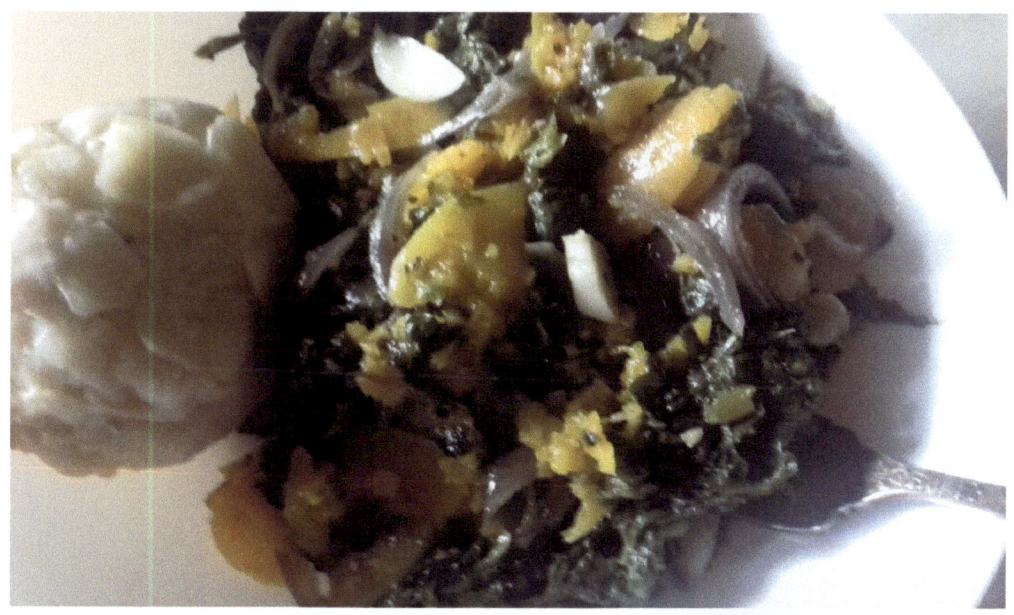

Young herring fresh food plate

place 2 herring fillets on a plate with
1 handful of arugula washed
3 slices of beet   peeled
Sauerkraut   or other fresh food of your choice &

      1 whole-grain roll

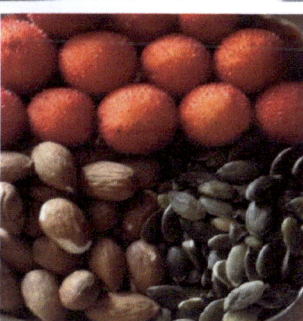

Raw food (enzymes) before every cooked meal!

I'd eat these young herrings any time of the day. In my youth, sometimes as a hangover breakfast. The Holland maties are very mild and hardly salty. The name may originate from the Dutch word for girl "Meisje".

Paprika curry with rice

1 onion   dice finely; sautée in a deep pan with
2-3 tbsp coconut oil grate or press and add
2-3 gloves of garlic cut
1-2 peppers   in strips and add them; cut and add

200 g mushrooms	slice, add and steam for 8 minutes; blend
2 tsp curry powder	
1 tsp sweet paprika powder and	
3 sprigs of parsley	chopped, stir in some coconut milk; fill up with
1 cup of coconut milk	and put it in the pan; boil briefly and remove from the fire; bring 2 cups water to a boil in a deep pan; add
1 cup Basmati rice	and cook on a low flame for about 20 minutes; the less water you take in, the more valuable nutrients you retain;

because when cooking, they come out of the rice and end up in the water. Better to proceed tactically with temperature and time than to lose nutrients!

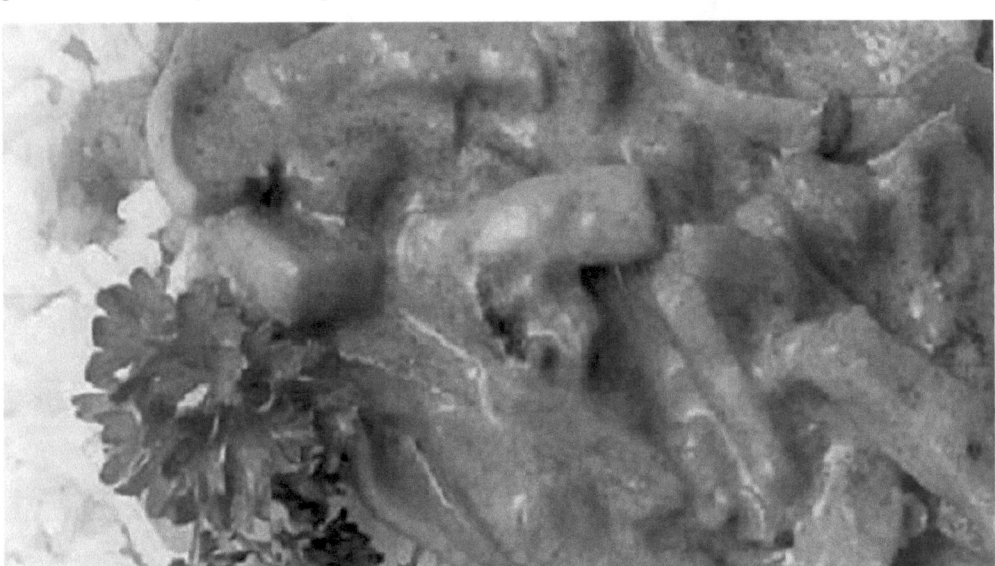

Pizza American style

1 ½ cups spelt whole-grain flour mix well with	
½ tsp Himalayan salt and	and
½ tsp baking soda	with 1 cup lukewarm water; add
2 tbsp olive oil	and quickly work into a smooth dough
	For the topping, mix some tomato paste with water

and oregano or an Italian herb mixture and spread on the pizza dough. Bake at 180° for approx. 20 minutes. I usually bake or cook by smell; once it starts smelling good, the dish is usually edible

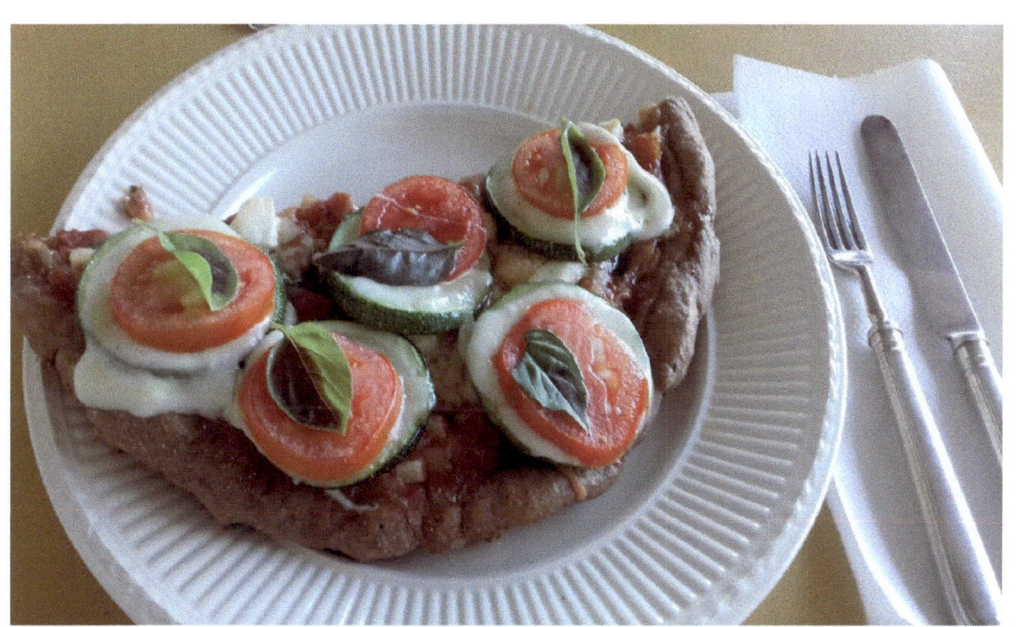

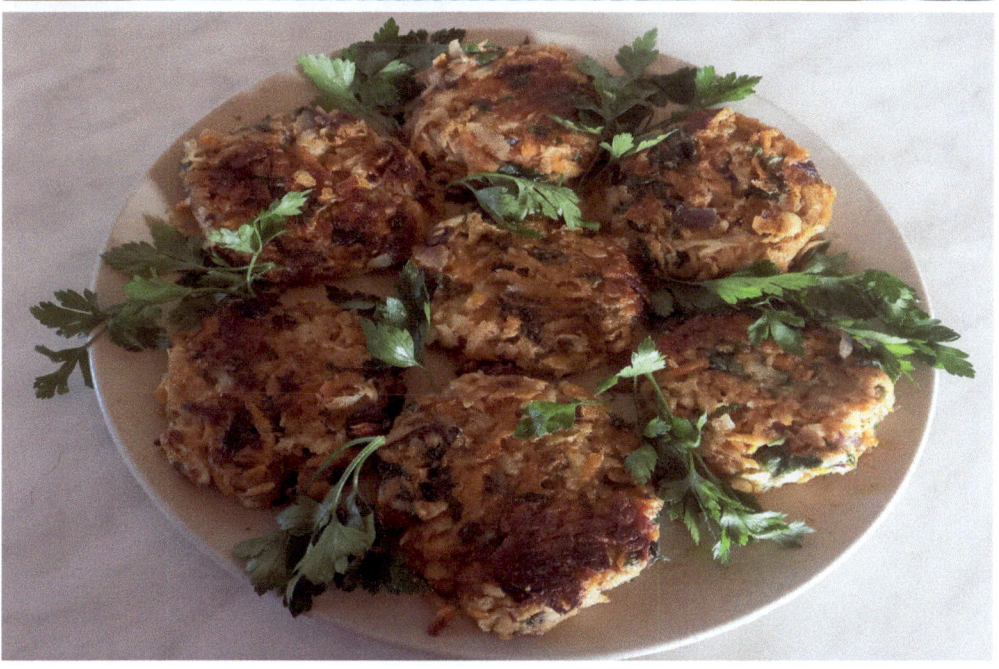

93

Radish Patties

½ radish	peel and grate
½ teaspoon of salt	mix in and leave for 8 minutes; cut
1 small red onion	into small cubes; wash and chop
½ bunch of parsley	peel and grate
4-5 potatoes	squeeze the liquid out in a cloth and mix the potatoes together with the squeezed out radish in a bowl; add
3 tbsp spelt flour	and the parsley as well as some salt
1 pinch grated nutmeg	and pepper from the mill, mix well, pour in the hot dough with a large spoon; add rapeseed oil, form into patties and bake from both sides

Salad over baked egg

2 slices of bread	fry 2 organic eggs to taste; butter the bread or grease them with olive oil and top with cucumber, tomato slices or green stuff

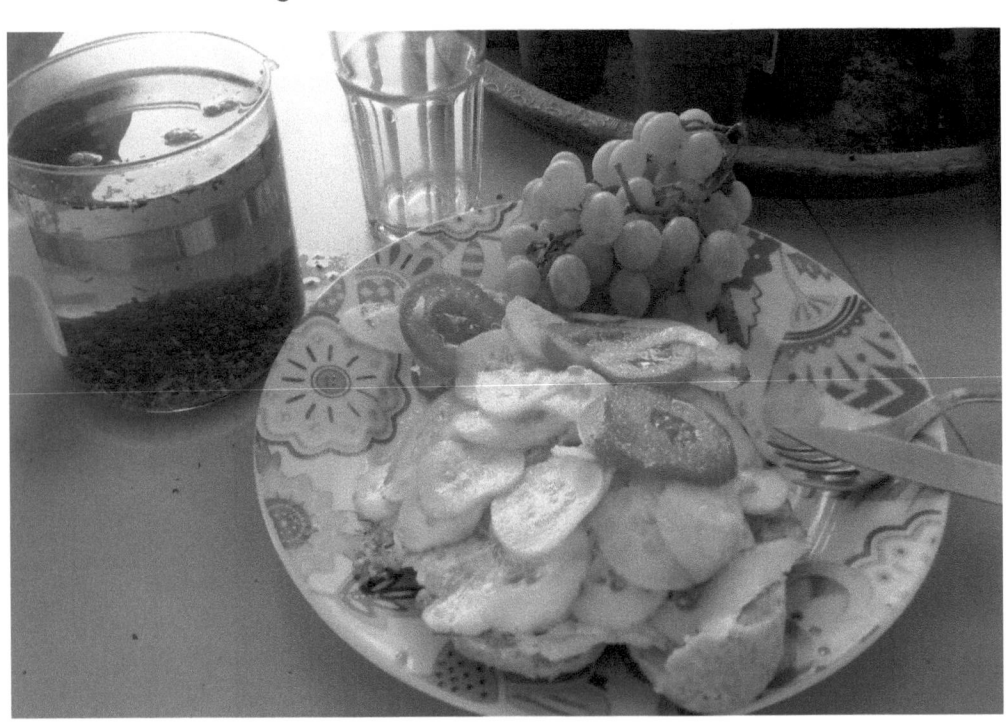

Sauerkraut bread

2 cups wholemeal spelt flour mix well with

1 cup sauerkraut

1 tsp ground juniper berries

1 tsp salt

1 tsp baking soda   add

 tbsp of apple cider vinegar and enough water to form a smooth dough; form a ball
and put it in a flour-dusted casserole or deep pan with
a lid; bake on a low flame for approx. 35 minutes

Shiitake mushrooms with sweet potatoes and spinach

2 cups spinach leaves   cook with

2 cups shiitake mushrooms   and

1 lg sweet potato   (wash well; brush if necessary) in

a little water   and

½ vegetable broth cube   on a low heat for 8 minutes; season with

2 tbsp organic olive oil   and spices of your choice; as light food
no further spices are necessary; otherwise, I first fry

1 red onion and 2 sliced garlic cloves in olive or colza oil and add the above
ingredients; for good digestion and protecting the pancreas, I usually eat papaya
and nuts (food enzymes) before a cooked meal

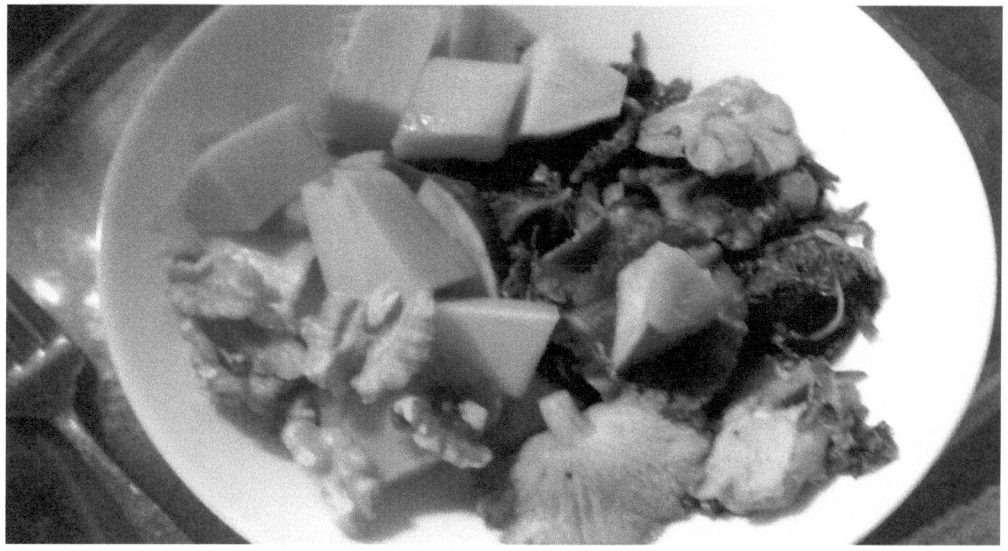

Shiitake mushrooms with mung bean sprouts

1 onion	slice and sauté; add
2 garlic cloves	crushed; wash and add
200 g shiitake mushrooms	wash and fold in
100 g mung bean sprouts	season with
1 tsp turmeric and/or ginger and	
fresh herbs	of your choice to taste; serve with basmati rice

Zucchini boats

2 zucchini	wash well; remove the stalk, cut in half lengthwise; with a tablespoon remove the core, scrape out and cut into small pieces; finely dice
1 lg onion	peel and finely dice
1 tomato	grate 3 garlic cloves very finely or press them; mix with
200 g cheese	(preferably fresh crumbly goat cheese); season with
salt & pepper	from the mill and herbs of your choice; fill in the boats and bake for 25 minutes at medium heat

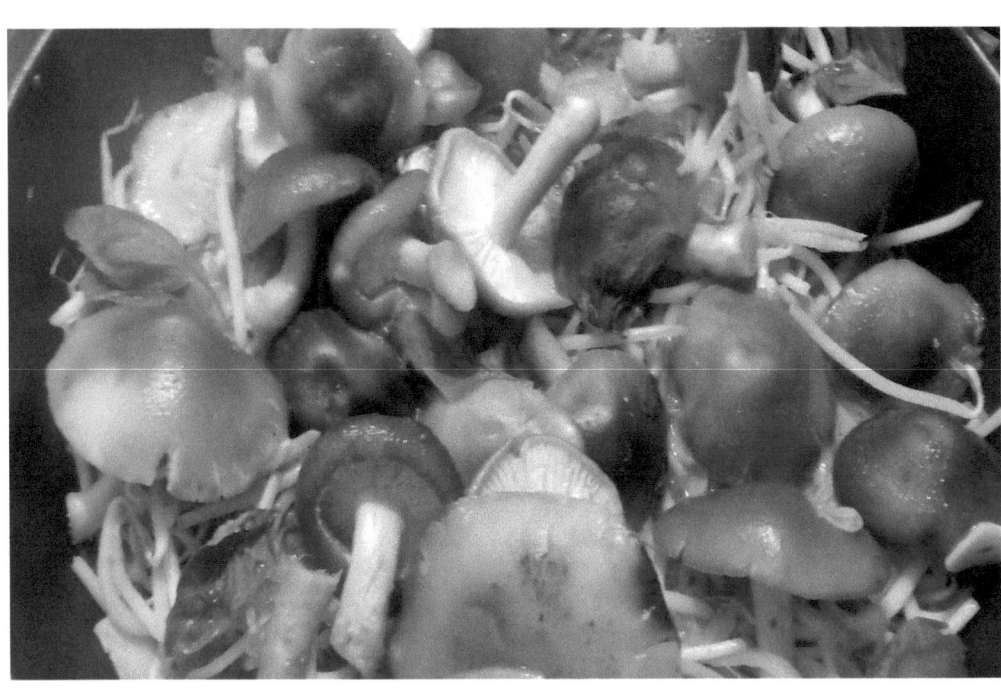

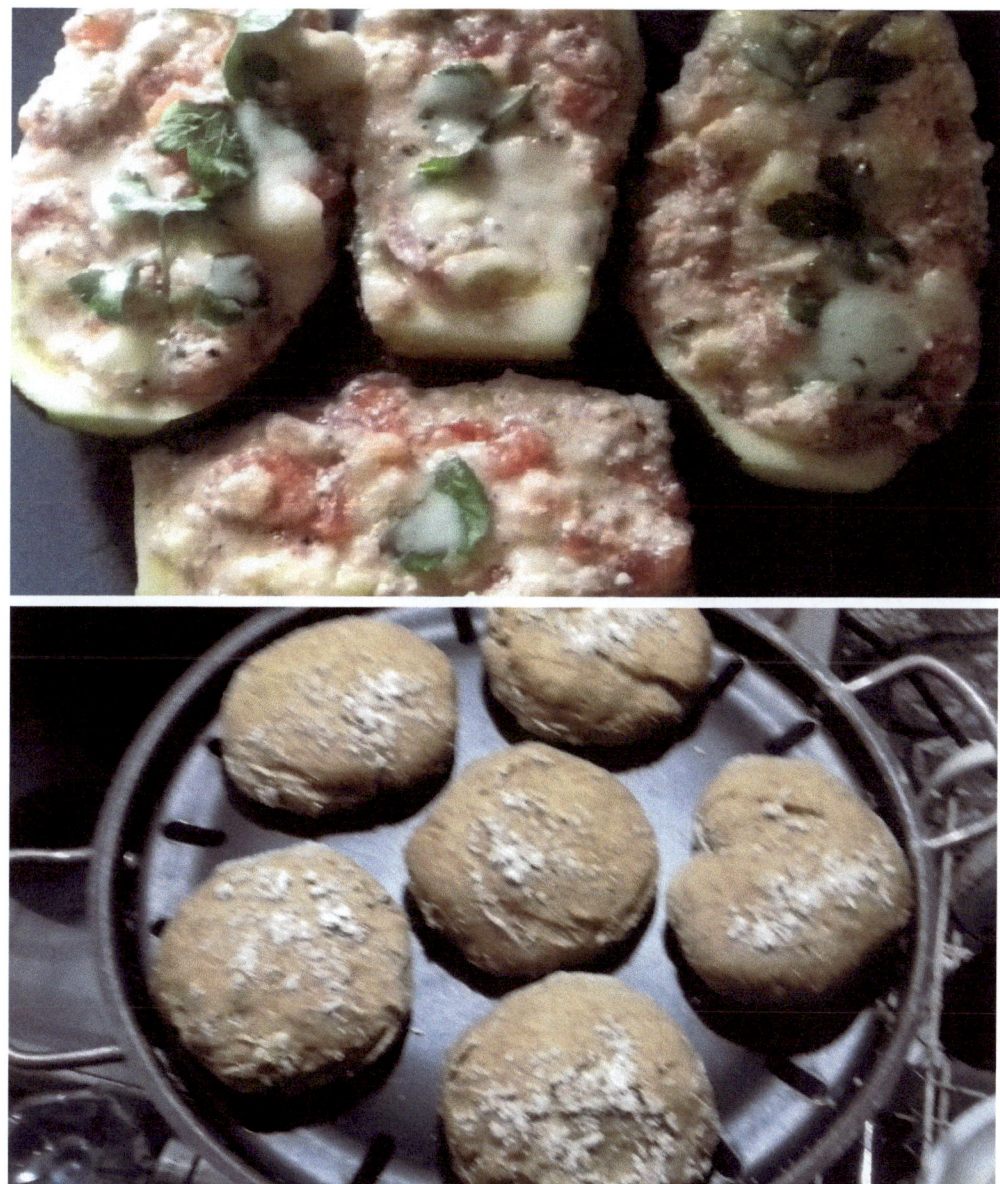

You can enjoy these spelt buns in 30 minutes. Mix about 2 ½ cups of flour with 1 level tsp of salt, 1 heaped tsp of baking soda, 3 tbsp of apple cider vinegar and about 1 cup of water to form a dough; form 6 rolls, and bake at approximately 160° 25 min. Here, in an Italian pan for 25 min., on low heat.

Closing remarks and thanks

The so-called coincidences are piling up again. It happens more when I'm about to finish a book. For example, I thought about what to write in the concluding remarks of the German edition. On the next day, I got an e-mail from Hans Würtz. He told me that, two months ago, his neighbor asked him for advice. His little dog of 13 years had abdominal cancer. One could feel and see the growth. Mercedes was very weak. The vet said she had a maximum of 10 days to live.

Hans said to his neighbor: "Put the hard ferrite plate measuring 15 cm x 10 cm x 2 cm that I gave you years ago in the sleeping basket of the little Mercedes. Put a blanket over the magnet. Thus the bitch does not lie so hard. The magnetic plate must point with the physical south pole to her abdomen. Fifteen years ago, for your mother-in-law's throat cancer treatment, I gave you one of my magnetic pulsers, which works according to the pulse scheme according to Dr Robert C. Beck. Your mother-in-law was cured and is now 90 years old. You also use this magnetic pulser every day on the small Mercedes in the abdominal area."

On Oct 5th, Hans met his neighbor again and asked him: "How is your little dog?" He said: "Mercedes is very jolly and often frolics around with the big dog.

No sign of illness anymore!"

And further explained Dipl.-Ing. Johann Würtz:
Every hand movement, every step we take, only works with electricity. Just like every thought we form. The functional processes of the organs are unthinkable without electricity and, of course, magnetism.

What is chemistry? What is biochemistry? It's electron physics!

Magnetic applications are electron spin applications with their left- and right-rotating torsion fields and thus also reach the area of the transcendent information level (nothing esoteric). They are part of the MAGNETO - ELECTRICAL MEDICINE (MEM) and are likely to transform future medicine from health, therapeutic, political and socio-economic perspectives. There will be a slow but steady change from medication with chemical substances to inexpensive treatment methods with few or no side effects and substance-free. Ultimately, all areas of medicine will experience a paradigm shift, including neurology, psychiatry, and the treatment of addiction and sex offenders. That opens up a broad field that urgently needs research".

If you want to know more about it, visit the Dipl.-Ing. Johann Würtz website: *wuertz-systems.jimdo.com/2018/08/23/electromagnetic-waves*

Apropos, if you like to reach my website, it is now also necessary to enter marianne-e-meyer.jimdo.com. Because before my vacation, I had commissioned the transfer to a cheaper webmaster. But when I came back from France, marianne-e-meyer.com no longer worked. Because I sold more books this quarter than before, I'll save on costs a for webmaster.

Speaking of the book, this one is also about magnetoelectric medicine, in much more detail in *WATER CONNECTS THE WORLDS.*

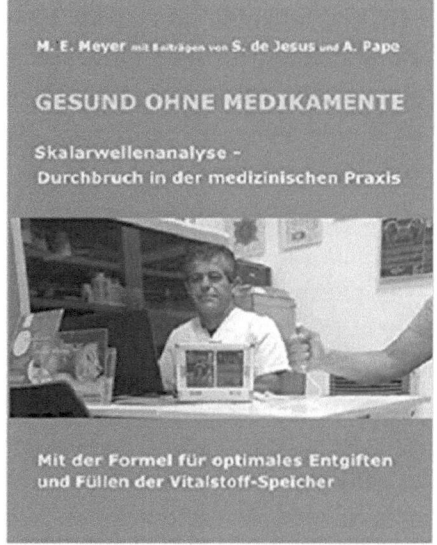

A breakthrough in medical diagnostics and therapy has been achieved. *GESUND OHNE MEDIKAMENTE* (Healthy without Medications) informs you about the communication of the cells and how undreamt-of healing chances open up to you via magnetic scalar waves. It is possible to turn back the biological clock.

Supplementing lacking micro-nutrients and a corresponding change in diet is the beginning of the rejuvenation cure.

In the early 1970s, Russia developed scalar wave analysis to monitor the health status of its cosmonauts in space. In Israel and the USA, the epochal device that works with scalar waves, which Nikola Tesla discovered more than a hundred years ago, is recognized by conventional medicine. Namely for the early detection of diseases and monitoring the progress of therapies. Around 200 parameters, including all blood values and harmful substances in the body or allergies, can be measured in around 1½ minutes without taking blood samples or lengthy diagnostic measures.

At this point, I would like to draw your attention to the *Innovative concepts for energy and health* congress taking place on June 18 / 19, 2022, in Stuttgart and the *Cosmic Energy in Technology and Health* congress on Sep 9 / 10, 2022, in Graz. Both are organized by Jupiter-Verlag, Schaffhausen/CH. Please refer to:

www.jupiter-verlag.ch/kongresse

But now to synchronicity: Don't you feel like it sometimes happens that strange coincidences suddenly start to pile up? Or you are suddenly in a hurry to get somewhere. They then meet a person who is otherwise never in that place at that time, and it turns out they have mutual acquaintances. Or they start a conversation with you and realize that they have problems, need help, give you a good tip or help you in some other way. Could it be that souls guide us via telepathy? Pay more attention to such guidance in the future. They show you that you are never alone. If you allow yourself to be led and see people you meet as an opportunity to grow, you are on the right track. Because when it's time for you to learn something, your teacher will soon be near you.

However, I don't sometimes understand how strange experiences are supposed to help me. Last October, e. g., I suddenly had the feeling that my deceased husband was present. I said: Peter, are you there? But nothing happened. A clairvoyant friend told me that Peter is sorry you can't hear him. Yes, maybe I should do a longer fasting cure again. On the following day, I woke up shortly before 6:00 a. m., and suddenly my cell phone lit up in the darkness. But it was off! At first, I thought have I forgotten to turn it off? But then the typical clicking noise asked me to enter my code. And things like this always happen when I'm in the final stages of a new book. Do our loved ones in the higher dimensions wish us luck when something comes up? Or did Peter want me to mention that in the closing words so that one or the other non-believer might turn inward or search for the meaning of their own life?

Could you do me a favor? If you have an exam coming up or a special event like a funeral, wedding, or birth, write down anything that strikes you as odd, especially if it has to do with electricity, because the spiritual world can connect with us via electricity. That has also shown a message from Toulouse Lautrec from 1981, channelled by the medium Luiz Antonio Gasparetto (see also p. 70).
https://www.youtube.com/watch?v=bWpc71VKiDI

I thank you in advance for your experiences, preferably via e-mail: drmarian-neemeyer @ gmail.com

Speaking of thanking: what's the saying? Nobody writes a book alone. I would therefore like to thank the following people for their suggestions, encouragement, help and ideas: Johann Würtz, Inge and Adolf Schneider, Sergio de Jesus, Wolfgang Meyer, Halima Neumann, Barbara Simonsohn, Renate Janzen, Brigitte Simon, Hedwig Müller, Ilona Brugger, Maurits Hagenaar and in addition to my late husband, all other participants from the sphere to which we will all return one day.

My special thanks go to Jeannette Forrer and other Deynique beauticians and naturopaths featured in my book *SO BEKOMMEN SIE IHR FETT WEG*. Thanks further go to Bob Hartmann, to whom I owe numerous interviews and seminars in which I learned that health and beauty are not just a question of consistent body care.

I would also like to thank *Grammarly* for its markedly well-done service.

I keep hearing from the glorifiers of modern medicine that we are now living longer than we used to. That's not correct. The average lifespan increased because infant mortality decreased. Statistically speaking, the high mortality rate at birth and infant mortality due to poor hygiene and malnutrition has exceedingly reduced life expectancy.

The disease industry has always wanted our best: our money. If you want to learn more about how medical professionals have always put their self-interests ahead of the patient's well-being under the guise of supposed scientific knowledge, here are a few links:

https://www.ncbi.nlm.nih.gov/pmc/articles/PMC1125506/

https://www.amazon.com/Strange-Medicine-Shocking-History-Practices/dp/0399159959

https://www.youtube.com/watch?v=MtAjIG45O64

IMPORTANT: Unless someone can find a living will, I'd better mention in every book that without the prospect of living or dying with dignity, I don't want to be artificially fed, have surgery, or receive chemotherapy.

Literatur

Aucoin M et al: The effect of Echinacea spp. on the prevention or treatment of COVID-19 and other respiratory tract infections in humans: A rapid review. Adv Integr Med 2020; Dec; 7(4): 203–217

Biesalski HK: Vitamin D deficiency and co-morbidities in COVID-19 patients – A fatal relationship? Nfs Journal. 2020 Aug; 20: 10–21

Bode AM et al.: The Amazing and Mighty Ginger. In: Herbal Medicine: Biomolecular and Clinical Aspects. 2nd edition. Boca Raton (FL): CRC Press/Taylor & Francis; 2011. Chapter 7.

Bodin J et al.: Vitamin D Deficiency is Associated with Increased Use of Antimicrobials among Pre-school Girls in Ethiopia. Nutrients 2019 Mar 7;11(3)

Bongo GN et al.: Aloe Vera (L.) Burm. F. as a Potential Anti-COVID-19 Plant: A Mini-review of Its Antiviral Activity. European Journal of Medicinal Plants · May 2020 DOI: 10.9734/ejmp/2020/v31i830261

Bouderbala H et al.: Anti-obesogenic effect of apple cider vinegar in rats subjected to a high fat diet. Ann Cardiol Angeiol (Paris)
.2016 Jun;65(3):208-13.

Cannon M L et al.: In Vitro Analysis of the Anti-viral Potential of nasal spray constituents against SARS-CoV-2,doi: https://doi.org/10.1101/2020.12.02.408575

Chaix et al.: Epigenetic clock analysis in long-term meditators. Psychoneuroendocrinology. 2017 Nov; 85:210-214

Chang JS et al.: Fresh ginger (Zingiber officinale) has anti-viral activity against human respiratory syncytial virus in human resp tract cell lines. J Ethnopharmacol. 2013 Jan 9;145 (1): 146-51

Chen, YH et al.: Well-tolerated Spirulina extract inhibits influenza virus replication and reduces virus-induced mortality. Sci Rep 2016; 6: 24253

Di Pierro, F et al.: Possible Therapeutic Effects of Adjuvant Quercetin Supplementation Against Early-Stage COVID-19 Infection: A Prospective, Randomized, Controlled, and Open-Label Study. Int J GenMed. 2021; 14: 2359–2366

Enshaieh S et al.: The efficacy of 5% topical tea tree oil gel in mild to moderate acne vulgaris: a randomized, double-blind placebo-controlled study. Indian J Dermatol Venereol Leprol. Jan-Feb 2007;73(1):22-5.

Felten, DL: „Psychosomatic Medicine", Vol. 42 (1980)6

Fitzgerald, Karen N.: Younger You: Reduce Your Bio Age and Live Longer, Better, Paris 2022

Gartz, Jochen: Wasserstoffperoxid: Das vergessene Heilmittel. Immenstadt 2014

Geesing, Hermann, „Immun-Training", München, 1990

Gordon M et al.: A placebo-controlled trial of the immune modulator, lentinan, in HIV-positive patients: a phase I/II trial. J Med. 1998;29(5-6):305-30

Grunewald F et al.: Effects of Birch Polypore Mushroom, Piptoporus betulinus (Agaricomycetes), the "Iceman's Fungus", on Human Immune Cells. Int J Med Mushrooms 2018;20(12):1135-1 1147.

Gustafson, KR et al.: AIDS-antiviral sulfolipids from cyanobacteria (blue-green algae) J Natl Cancer Inst. 1989 Aug 16;81(16):1254-8. doi: 10.1093/jnci/81.16.1254

Halima BH, Sonia G, Sarra K, Houda BJ, Fethi BS, Abdallah A.: Apple Cider Vinegar

Attenuates Oxidative Stress and Reduces the Risk of Obesity in High-Fat-Fed Male Wistar Rats. J Med Food. 2018 Jan;21(1):70-80.

Harunobu A, Nance DM: A randomized, double-blind, placebo-controlled, clinical study of the general effects of a standardized Lycium barbarum (Goji) Juice, GoChi. J Altern Complement Med. 2008 May;14(4):403-12

Hellwig MD, Maia A: A COVID-19 prophylaxis? Lower incidence associated with prophylactic administration of ivermectin. 2021 Jan;57(1):106248.doi: 10.1016/j. Ijantimicag 2020.106248. Epub 2020 Nov 28.

Hiedra R et al.: The Use of IV vitamin C for patients with COVID-19: A single center observational study. *Expert Rev. Anti-Infect. Ther.* 2020;18:1259–1261

Jaskulska A et al.: Thapsigargin, a tumor promoter, discharges intracellular Ca2+ stores by specific inhibition of the endoplasmic reticulum Ca2(+)-ATPase. Proc Natl Acas Sci USA.1990 Apr; 87(7): 2466–2470

Jeremiah SS et al.: Potent antiviral effect of silver nanoparticles on SARS-CoV-2. Biochem Biophys Res Commun. 2020 Nov 26;533(1):195-200

Kang Y et al.: Preventive effects of Goji berry on dextran-sulfate-sodium-induced colitis in mice. J Nutr Biochem. 2017 Feb:4070-76

König, Ralf: Vervirte Zeiten

Kreutz G et al.: Effects of choir singing or listening on secretory immunoglobulin A, cortisol, and emotional state. J Behav Med. 2004 Dec;27(6):623-35

Kreutzer, Martin, Anne Larsen: Mit der richtigen Ernährung heimliche Entzündungen bekämpfen. Riva-Verlag 2018

Kuchta A et al.: The effect of Cistus incanus herbal tea supplementation on oxidative stress markers and lipid profile in healthy adults. Cardiol J. 2019 Mar 26.doi: 10.5603/CJ. 2019.0028

Kumar R et al.: Putative roles of vitamin D in modulating immune response and immunopathology associated with COVID-19. Virus Res. 2021 Jan 15;292:19823

Langguth, Veronik: Atmen Sie sich gesund: Mit Fingerdruckpunkten den heilsamen Atem aktivieren. München 2019

Lindequist U et al.: The Pharmacological Potential of Mushrooms. Evid Based Complement Alternat Med. 2005 Sep; 2(3): 285–299

Lopresti AL, Drummond PD, Smith SJ: A Randomized, Double-Blind, Placebo-Controlled, Crossover Study Examining the Hormonal and Vitality Effects of Ashwagandha (Withania somnifera) in Aging, Overweight Males. Am J Mens Health. Mar-Apr 2019;13(2):1557988319835985

Lopresti AL et al.: An investigation into the stress-relieving and pharmacological actions of an ashwagandha (Withania somnifera) extract: A randomized, double-blind, placebo-controlled study. Medicine (Baltimore). 2019 Sep;98(37):e17186

Mahli HK et al.: Tea tree oil gel for mild to moderate acne; a 12 week uncontrolled, open-label phase II pilot study.Australas J Dermatol. 2017 Aug;58(3):205-210

Martineau AR et al.: Vitamin D supplementation to prevent acute respiratory tract inf ections: systematic review and meta-analysis of individual participant data. BMJ.2017 Feb 15;356:i658.doi: 10. 1136/bmj. I6583

103

Matheusz G, Skwarlo-Sonta K: Mechanisms involved in the anti-inflammatory action of inhaled tea tree oil in mice. Exp Biol Med (Maywood).2007 Mar;232(3):420-6

Mentel R et al.: Virus inactivation by hydrogen peroxide. Vopr Virusol. Nov-Dec 1977;(6):731-3

Meyer, Marianne: Wasserkristalle: Botschaft der Seelen. Norderstedt 2021
  Cranberry Powerfruit, Norderstedt 2017
  Spirulina, Survival Food for a New Era. Norderstedt 2016

Mohd Yusof, YA: Gingerol and Its Role in Chronic Diseases. Adv Exp Med Biol. 2016; 2016;929:177-207

Moreira H et al.: Antioxidant and cancer chemopreventive activities of cistus and pomegranate polyphenols Acta Pol Pharm . 2017 Mar;74(2):688-698

Mota, ACLG et al: Antifungal Activity of Apple Cider Vinegar on Candida Species Involved in Denture Stomatitis. J Prosthodont. 2015 Jun;24(4):296-302.5

Mukerjee PK et al.: Phytochemical and therapeutic profile of *Aloe Vera*. J. Nat. Remedies. 2014;14:1–26.

Murphy EJ et al.: β-Glucan extracts from the same edible shiitake mushroom Lentinus edodes produce differential in-vitro immunomodulatory and pulmonary cytoprotective effects - Implications for coronavirus disease (COVID-19) immunotherapies. Sci Total Environ. 2020 Aug 25;732:139330

Neumann, Halima: Stop der Azidose, Allergien und Haarausfall, Fürhoff/Spira Verde 2008

Obeta MU: Anti-COVID-19 Properties of Ginger (Zingiber officinale) assisted Enugu – Nigerian People During the Pandemic. J BacteriolInfectDis. 2020;S(3):5

Park WH: Hydrogen peroxide inhibits the growth of lung cancer cells via the induction of cell death and G1-phase arrest. Oncol Rep. 2018 Sep;40(3):1787-1794

Pentón-Rol G et al.: C-Phycocyanin-derived Phycocyanobilin as a Potential Nutraceutical Approach for Major Neurodegenerative Disorders and COVID-19-induced Damage to the Nervous System. Curr Neuropharmacol. 2021 Apr 8.

Ratha SK et al.: Prospective options of algae-derived nutraceuticals as supplements to combat COVID-19 and human coronavirus diseases. Nutrition 2021 Mar; 83: 111089

Rauwald HW et al.: Labdanum and Labdanes of Cistus creticus and C. ladanifer: Anti-Borelia activity and its phytochemical profiling.Phytomedicine. 2019 Jul;60:152977

Simons, Peter Carl: Aloe Vera 6.000 Jahre Medizingeschichte können sich nicht irren. Norderstedt 2015

Signer, J. et al.:In vitro virucidal activity of Echinaforce®, an *Echinacea purpurea* preparation, against coronaviruses, including common cold coronavirus 229E and SARS-CoV-2. Virology Journal (2020) 17:136

Simonsohn, Barbara: Stevia, sündhaft süß und urgesund, Aitrang 2010

Singh N et al.: An Overview on Ashwagandha: A Rasayana (Rejuvenator) of Ayurveda. Afr J Tradit Complement Altern Med. 2011; 8(5 Suppl): 208–213

Spyridopoulou K et al.: Extraction, Chemical Composition, and Anticancer Potential of Origanum onites L. Essential Oil. Molecules 2019 Jul; 24(14): 2612

Steiner-Ehrenberger, Doris: Antibiotika-Resistenz. In Lebe natürlich Magazin 1-21

Sullivan SE, Stevenson CW, Laviolette SR: Could Cannabidiol Be a Treatment for Coronavirus Disease-19-Related Anxiety Disorders? Cannabis Cannabinoid Res Res. 2021 Feb 12;6(1):7-18

Tan XL et al: Polyporus umbellatus inhibited tumor cell proliferation and promoted tumor cell apoptosis by down-regulating AKT in breast cancer. Biomed Pharmacother. 2016 Oct;83:526-535

Thimmulappa RK et al.: Antiviral and immunomodulatory activity of curcumin: A case for prophylactic therapy for COVID-19. Heliyon. 2021 Feb;7(2):e06350

Tzachor A et al.: Photosynthetically Controlled Spirulina, but Not Solar Spirulina, Inhibits TNF-α Secretion: Potential Implications for COVID-19-Related Cytokine Storm Therapy. Mar Biotechnol (NY). 2021 Feb;23(1):149-155

Vincent MJ et al.: Chloroquine is a potent inhibitor of SARS coronavirus infection and spread. Virol J 2005; 2: 69

Weidner, Christopher, Wunderpflanze Zistrose: Die unglaublichen Heilerfolge mit Cystus Rottenburg 2011

Weiss, EI et al.: Cranberry juice constituents affect influenza virus adhesion and infectivity. Antiviral Res.2005 Apr;66(1):9-12

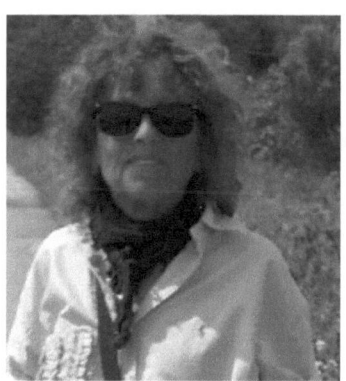

Marianne Erika Meyer, PhD

Helping people get well has always been my dream. So I first worked as a medical assistant. Later, while I studied pedagogy at the University in Frankfurt, I visied children suffering from spasticity and cancer and older people in a residential complex for the elderly in Frankfurt.

I also gave Reiki to Louise Hays AIDS support group members in the USA for seven years. Through the latter work, the thesis in nutritional science *strengthen the immune system with Spirulina platensis* developed as my doctoral.

In 1997, living in Germany again, I published my results in books from Windpferd Verlag. Via lectures and thanks to Dr Hittich, who gave away fifty thousand copies of my bestseller *Spirulina, das blaugrüne Wunder* (the blue-green miracle) to his customers as a special edition, I made the beneficial algae known in Europe.

Until years ago, I worked with young people with behavioral problems in Portugal. After my husband died, I edited books for Jim Humble Publishing for two years. Currently, I daily hike in the mountains, rescuing free-roaming animals. And until the coronavirus emerged, I sang alongside my paperwork in the EAISC choir, mostly in multi-generational and senior citizen centers. Now I guess I have to look for a choir allowing non-vaccinated members.

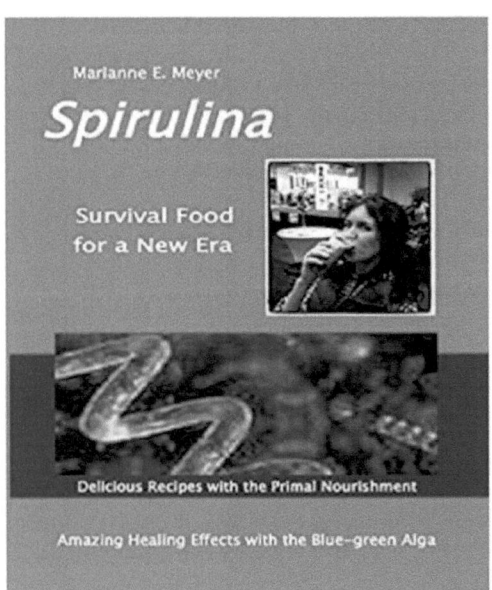

Marianne E. Meyer

Spirulina

Survival Food for a New Era

Delicious Recipes with the Primal Nourishment

Amazing Healing Effects with the Blue-green Alga

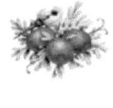

Marianne E. Meyer

CRANBERRY POWER FRUIT

Handbook to the Methuselah Berry

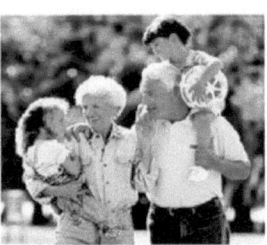

Sensational Healing Successes and Delicious Recipes for the Healthy Kitchen

We all need Spirulina. Why? Because of infertile soils, we can hardly get energy from our food. The blue-green alga is concentrated solar power since it contains all the colors of the spectrum and thus all frequencies of light, just like the water of Lourdes.

Marianne Erika Meyer introduced "Spirulina, das blaugrüne Wunder" (the blue-green miracle) via her same-named German bestseller and an appearance on Prime TV in German-speaking Europe and Russia. Evermore folks supplement their diets with beneficial protein food. And dentists use it progressively for discharging amalgam and other toxins.

Stunning studies & reports around the globe prove: With Spirulina, we strengthen our immune system and stand up to pain, depression, diabetes, MS, cataracts, allergies, anemia, arthritis, liver fibrosis, and Parkinson's disease, and even AIDS and cancer.

In the illustrated book with delicious recipes, the PhD nutritionist covered each chapter in note form and highlighted crucial parts.

ISBN 978-3734728525 104 p. 17x22cm €7,99

This revised translation of the first practical cranberry handbook informs comprehensive on the rejuvenating fruit.

The expert for natural remedies shows how cranberry is indispensable as natural health care helper. Cranberry prevents the adhesion of bacteria for bladder infections, acute cystitis, and urinary tract infections. It may even represent a promising co-adjuvant for preventing and treating COVID-19. Due to its antithrombotic and anti-inflammatory properties, its resveratrol expects to reduce COVID-19-associated mortality.

Cranberry's best-established medical applications are preventing and treating bacterial infections of the urinary tract, the gastric mucosa and the oral cavity.

This work demonstrates the potential of preventing and curing some 80% of all health problems, including cardiovascular diseases (especially atherosclerosis), rheumatoid arthritis and cancer. We can turn back the clock, reversing premature aging symptoms.

Delicious recipes from Marianne Meyer's health kitchen and trendy cocktails complete the book with the red round power fruit.

ISBN 978-3743181595 104 p. 17x22cm €7,99

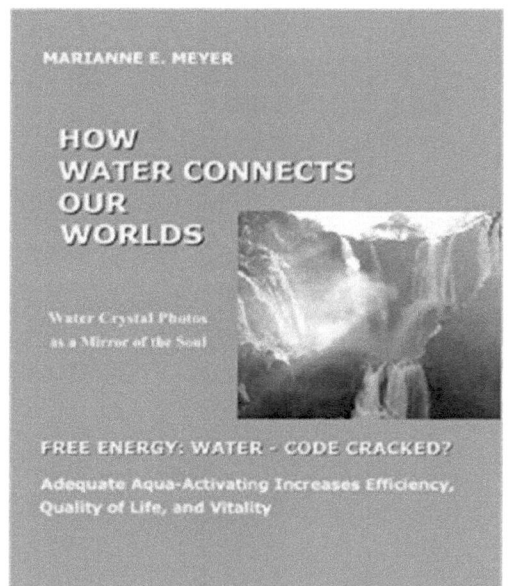

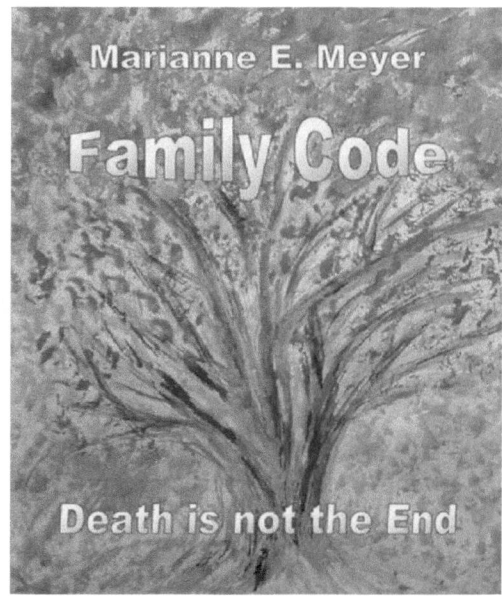

Our body and everything around us are vibrating water that responds to voices, moods and music. The Japanese water researcher Masaru Emoto discovered water molecules changing according to the sounds exposed.

In cooperation with the water artist Ernst Braun, Marianne Meyer found out who realizes the water art. She explains her research results comprehensible, using many partly colored water crystal photos in different tests.

The book leads you on the path into the depths of life and reveals the secret in our genes. By embracing our shadows and realizing how much our trained way of thinking influences us, fear no longer has to impair our mental power in the future. Another content is the principle of shaping our reality by making it clear to ourselves what we want. What we do to make ourselves and others happy is precisely what makes us happy.

The reader also will find disturbing facts about the quality of commercial and tap waters. The author advises using activating water adequately.

Ultimately, the author introduces free energy researchers and their technologies. She also shows what to do, so space energy can soon flow in all households.

ISBN 978-3734736919 **104 p. 17x22cm €7,99**

In this captivating autobiographical novel, we take part in the author's exciting intercontinental life. It becomes clear that we are all connected and that families have had their value systems for generations.

This code of own rules, idioms and communication styles expresses even when family members live on different continents without knowing each other.

The book represents a bridge that connects the realm of the living and that of the dead. It shows there is no guilt, chance or luck, only cause and effect, which may be many centuries and incarnations apart. Luck, bad luck and chance are just terms for the law that is not yet recognized. And if you don't learn, you suffer. The only thing that remains is what connects the worlds, the only meaning of life: LOVE.

Reader I. B.G.: "The book conveys crystal clear lived spirituality and belongs in every household."

At BoD or or other online book stores, you can read part of the book, but for cosmic plus points, it is better to order it from the local bookseller.

ISBN 978-3741282331 **184 p. 17x22 cm €8.98**

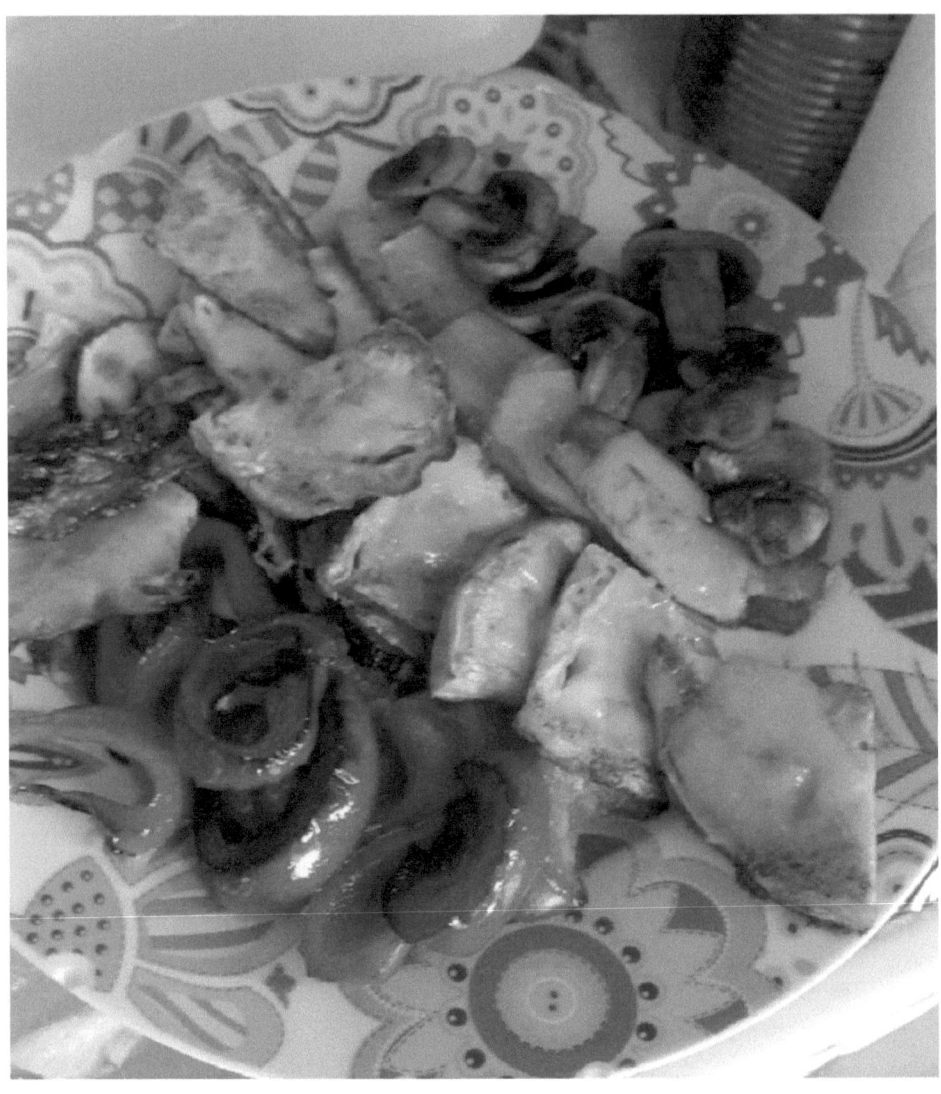

After 4 p. m. it is better not to eat raw vegetables, as they often cause bloating. Steaming would be perfect, but this appetizer platter would also be a healthy snack.